Also by the American Cancer Society

Prostate Cancer
Women and Cancer

American Cancer Society
COLORECTAL CANCER

American Cancer Society

COLORECTAL CANCER

*A Thorough and Compassionate
Resource for Patients and
Their Families*

Bernard Levin, M.D.

Editorial Project Director
Ron Schaumburg

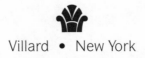

Villard • New York

The patients described in the book are composites based on actual cases from Dr. Levin's practice. All patient names and identifying details—ages, occupations, places of residence, and so on—have been altered to protect confidentiality. In some cases, details from two or more cases have been combined so as to make the point in a single story. The cases are for illustrative purposes only. While they are based on Dr. Levin's clinical experiences and inspired by real individuals, in no instance is it possible to identify an actual patient based on any detail as given.

*To Ronnie, Adam, and Katie for their love,
patience, and support*

Acknowledgments

We are pleased to have had the full support of the American Cancer Society (ACS) in the development of this book. Without the commitment of the ACS, and the moral support of the Advisory Group on Colorectal Cancer, what you have before you would not be possible. I would like to thank Harmon Eyre, M.D., vice president of the American Cancer Society National Home Office, whose unwavering enthusiasm and encouragement has supported us all. Dr. Robert Smith, Director of Cancer Screening for the American Cancer Society, has been a perpetual source of support and good advice.

I would especially like to thank the members of the ACS Advisory Group on Colorectal Cancer who provided moral support, including Dr. Tim Byers, Dr. Donald Anthony, Dr. Jerome DeCosse, Dr. Gerald Dodd, Dr. Charles Erlichman, Dr. Stanley Hamilton, Debra Jackson, Dr. Edward Mansour, Dr. Bruce Minsky, Dr. Richard Nelson, Gloria Peterson, Ph.D., Dr. Stan Riepe, Dr. Mary Elizabeth Roth, Dr. David Rothenberger, Dr. Mary Simmonds, and Marion Nadel, Ph.D.

I would also like to acknowledge the help that I have received over the years from numerous colleagues and patients who have provided inspiration and wisdom for the material within these pages. Although the patient stories in this book are drawn from actual cases and interviews, details and names have been changed and no association between any story and the names should be inferred.

Thanks to Dr. Ted Gansler and his staff at ACS for reviewing and editing the clinical material in the book; Jeff Clements, database researcher, for his countless hours of research; and Emily Pualwan, publishing director, and Jennifer Miller, production coordinator, for moving the project through its many steps to completion. Thanks to the following individuals: Barbara Lowenstein of Lowenstein and Associates, the project's literary agent, and her staff; Mollie Doyle, our editor at Villard Books; and Charles Boyter for his prompt and professional production of the illustrations. I am also most appreciative of all the efforts of my assistants, Rosanne Lemon and Nora Durham.

Finally, a special thanks to Ron Schaumburg, the meticulous project director and editorial advisor, whose efforts were essential in the success of this book. I couldn't praise him highly enough.

Contents

American Cancer Society
COLORECTAL CANCER

Chapter 1

Overview

Recently, I had the happy task of reporting some good news to a patient I'll call Louise.* Now sixty-three years old, Louise is a vibrant, active woman. Three times a grandmother, she works part-time at a radio station not far from my practice at the University of Texas M. D. Anderson Cancer Center, a leading treatment and research facility in Houston. Every Saturday night, Louise and her husband go square dancing at a local community center.

A few years ago, though, Louise heard some news that did not make her feel much like dancing.

Because of a change in her insurance coverage, Louise went to see a new internist for her routine annual physical examination. This alert doctor noted that she was over the age of fifty, the time of life when the risk of cancer of the colon and rectum begins to increase. He suggested that she should consider having a sigmoidoscopy—a procedure in which the physician uses a viewing tube to look for possible problems in the lower part of the intestine. Although she felt perfectly fine, she was eager to do what was best for her health, so she agreed.

During the procedure, the physician noticed the presence of a few unusual growths in the lining of the colon. These growths, called *polyps*, looked like tiny mushrooms, with slender stalks

---

* To ensure privacy, patients' names and personal descriptions have been changed.

leading to caps. Most polyps are completely harmless, but, over time, a small percentage of them may turn into cancer. The sigmoidoscope is not employed to examine the entire colon, where other polyps may possibly grow. The doctor reassured Louise that she was in no immediate danger, but he urged her to see a specialist in digestive problems, who would want to take a closer look. That's when she made an appointment with me.

During the exam, I used a device called a colonoscope, which allowed me to examine the entire length of her large intestine. I spotted several additional polyps growing in a region that the sigmoidoscope, because of its shorter length, could not have revealed. Using a special instrument, I snipped off these growths and sent them to a laboratory for analysis.

A pathologist—a physician who looks at tissue samples under a microscope—studied the tissue. The lab report confirmed what I had suspected: the cells of the tissue contained the beginning signs of cancer. However, we had caught the problem in time. The cancer existed only in the tip of one of the polyps; it had not yet spread into the stalks, nor had it penetrated other layers of the intestine.

When I told Louise that we had found cancer in her colon, she was surprised and, needless to say, scared. "How could I have cancer?" she asked. "I feel just fine. I don't feel anything is wrong." I explained that, in many cases, colon cancer causes no symptoms until it has reached the advanced stages, at which point a cure may not be possible.

I also pointed out that she was lucky. Because she had undergone a routine physical exam that included screening for cancer, her doctors had been able to spot the problem early and take appropriate action.

Still, I had to caution her that she wasn't completely out of the woods. The nature of colon cancer is such that, even after growths like Louise's are removed, there's about a 40 percent chance that new ones may develop later in life. I asked Louise to come back in a year so that I could repeat the colonoscopy.

Louise kept that appointment, and, after the test, I could give her the reassuring news that no new polyps had developed.

Because polyps grow very slowly, I suggested that Louise should return in three years for a follow-up visit, which she did. That was a few weeks ago. She was delighted when I told her the good news: no new growths.

Louise will need to remain vigilant for the rest of her life. But because her cancer was diagnosed early, treated, and cured, she and her husband will enjoy many more nights of square dancing in the years to come.

As Louise found out, receiving a diagnosis of cancer is a frightening and disorienting experience. Dealing with the uncertainties of an unpredictable and potentially fatal illness, trying to understand the treatment options, navigating the maze of the health care system—all of these contribute to the burden of cancer.

Adding to the personal stress is the very nature of colorectal cancer. The disease develops within the digestive system and affects the organ through which the body eliminates solid waste. The process of diagnosing and treating the disease often involves the use of bowel-cleansing procedures (enemas) or devices inserted into the body through the anus. Such procedures, while usually not painful, can be uncomfortable, and people naturally find them unpleasant or embarrassing. Not surprisingly, these factors make people reluctant to take the steps necessary to detect colorectal cancer at an early stage, before symptoms develop, when the chances of cure are highest.

Although they are difficult to think about, these things are important for reducing the risk of colorectal cancer and for getting the right treatment if cancer is discovered. That's what this book is about. The message I want to convey is that colorectal cancer is one of the most preventable forms of cancer. As I will explain in Chapter 4, by making some basic changes in their lifestyle, most people can greatly improve their chances of avoiding the disease. Also, because of the way this cancer develops over time, detecting it early and treating it appropriately can mean an excellent chance of full recovery.

I am aware, however, that most people who read this book will probably do so because colorectal cancer has already been diagnosed in themselves or in someone they love. For those readers and their families, this book will explain what happens within the patient's body. I will describe the treatments available and will explain how a combination of therapies, lifestyle changes, and careful follow-up monitoring offers the best chance for dealing with the disease, preventing its recurrence, and living a normal life for as long as possible.

After Louise overcame the initial shock of having cancer diagnosed and treated, she adopted a positive attitude about her condition. As she put it, "I'm not dying from cancer — I'm living with it." For people who have colorectal cancer, that is an attitude I hope this book will foster.

It has often been said that knowledge is power. That is especially true when dealing with a serious medical illness such as colorectal cancer. The more you know, the smarter your choices will be, and the more power you will have over the disease, its treatment, and the outcome.

This introductory chapter will summarize the book's main themes. It is important to define what cancer is and to identify the parts of the body that are affected by colorectal cancer. Detailed information is given in Chapters 2 and 3. For now, a brief discussion will suffice.

Every organ in the body is made of up of millions of cells — tiny structures that carry out the tasks necessary to sustain life. Normally, cells reproduce themselves by dividing. The new cells replace old ones, which die and are broken down and removed from the body.

In cancer, however, something happens to change the way the cells reproduce. The abnormal cells multiply at a rapid and uncontrolled rate, crowding out the normal healthy cells. The cancerous cells collect in masses known as tumors. As the cancer progresses, it becomes more dangerous. A tumor can grow so large that it interferes with the function of an organ. In colorectal cancer, the tumor can block the passage of feces through the intestine. Cancerous cells can also penetrate the wall of the colon or rectum and invade other nearby organs or tissues.

In the most serious cases, cancer cells leave the tumor and travel to other locations in the body, where they can cause new tumors to grow. This process, called metastasis, is dangerous because it damages other organs, makes the disease more difficult to treat, and sharply increases the risk of disability or death. This is a key reason why prevention and early detection are so important. Because of the way colorectal cancer grows, it can usually be identified long before it can penetrate the intestine or travel to another location in the body.

The intestines are part of the system that digests the food we eat. After leaving the stomach, the partially digested food enters the small intestine, a narrow tube about twenty feet in length. A few hours later, the remaining solid matter passes into the large intestine (also called the large bowel), which is wider in diameter and about five or six feet in length.

The colon, which makes up about five-sixths of the large intestine, rises on the right side of the body, crosses over, and descends on the left. Its shape is somewhat like the letter M.

At the end of the colon is the rectum. About eight inches long, the rectum serves to contain waste matter (feces) just prior to a bowel movement (defecation). Although they have different functions, the colon and the rectum are often discussed together as the colorectum. Colorectal cancer refers to a cancer in either portion of the large bowel.

Waste matter that is being expelled from the body passes through the anal canal, a tube about two or three inches long. At the end of the canal is the anus, a muscular ring through which feces leave the body. Cancer that develops in the anus is different from colorectal cancer and requires a different approach to treatment.

The important point to remember about colorectal cancer is that it usually begins as a noncancerous collection of cells called polyps, which grow along the inner lining of the large intestine. If detected early, these polyps can be removed using a relatively minor surgical procedure. If left untreated, however, the harmless cells in a polyp may undergo a transformation and become cancerous. Even if the cancer is detected in this later stage, surgery can remove the polyps (and part or all of the colon if necessary) and prevent the disease from spreading to other sites in the body. (Chapter 3 gives more information about how colorectal cancer evolves in stages.)

WHAT CAUSES COLORECTAL CANCER?

The precise cause of colorectal cancer is not fully known. The most likely explanation is that, over time, several factors work together to cause cancer to develop. Evidence points to fat in the diet as one main source of the problem. Fat takes longer to digest than other nutrients. The process of breaking down fat can cause a kind of "residue" in the intestine, not unlike the soot and ash burning wood or coal can leave behind. When they accumulate, these byproducts of digestion appear to irritate or damage the cells in the colon, causing them to undergo abnormal or uncontrolled growth.

Eating fat also triggers the release of bile, a liquid secreted by the liver and stored in the gallbladder. Bile helps the digestion of fats. The more fat one eats, the more bile the body must produce. Bile is made up of a number of components, including water, bilirubin, cholesterol, and various bile acids. Some evidence suggests that the presence of excess bile, especially bile acids, may be a contributing factor in colorectal cancer.

The American diet is generally lower in vegetables and fruits than it should be. These important foods provide a number of elements and minerals that help the body function normally and, in the process, help protect cells against the cancer-causing effects of other compounds. A growing body of evidence indicates that these foods act as natural cancer preventives.

Vegetables and fruits also contain a substance called fiber, which gives structure to the cells of plant products. Fiber does not get broken down by the body during digestion; instead, it passes through virtually unchanged. Fiber may help prevent cancer by absorbing fat or by speeding up the rate at which fat passes through the intestine. Lack of fiber, especially in a diet high in fat, can contribute to the risk of the disease.

In a small percentage of cases, colorectal cancer is the result of genes passed on from generation to generation. There are two main types of hereditary colon cancer:

1. Familial adenomatous polyposis (FAP) is a genetic defect that causes the growth of hundreds or even thousands of polyps in the large intestine, usually beginning at an early age. The risk is very high—nearly 100 percent—that at least some of these polyps will develop into cancerous tumors.
2. Hereditary nonpolyposis colorectal cancer (HNPCC) does not cause the growth of large numbers of polyps, but it does involve a higher-than-average risk of cancer.

We cannot change our genetic makeup. However, people who know they are at risk because of a strong family history of colorectal cancer (for example, the disease has been diagnosed at a young age in at least three family members in two different generations) can undergo preventive surgery to remove the colon and stop the disease before it develops. More information about these conditions appears in Chapter 3.

WHAT ARE THE SYMPTOMS OF COLORECTAL CANCER?

Colorectal cancer may not cause any symptoms at all. The symptoms that do develop usually involve a change in bowel habits.

For example, some people experience recurring inability to have a bowel movement (constipation), or the opposite problem, frequent watery bowel movements (diarrhea). The stools that are passed may be narrower than usual. Other symptoms include blood in the stool, abdominal pain, or cramps. If the bleeding is severe, anemia can result, leading to weakness and fatigue. Anal cancer can cause bleeding, itching, pain, and the feeling that there is a growth in the tissue.

Such symptoms are not unique to colorectal cancer. They often accompany other diseases, especially those affecting the bowel, such as colitis or Crohn's disease. Anyone experiencing worrisome digestive or abdominal symptoms should see a doctor. Effective treatment begins with an accurate diagnosis.

WHO GETS COLORECTAL CANCER?

When scientists discuss the *incidence* of a disease, they mean the number of new cases diagnosed each year. Colorectal cancer has the fourth-highest incidence of all internal cancers.* The only internal cancers that occurs more often among women are breast and lung cancers. Among men, colorectal cancer is third in frequency, following lung cancer and cancer of the prostate gland.

The incidence of colorectal cancer has been decreasing in recent years. In 1990, there were 142,300 new cases of colorectal cancer, compared to 139,000 in 1994 and an estimated 131,600 cases in 1998. Of these, 95,600 will involve the colon, and 36,600 will be cancer of the rectum. (Anal cancer is much less common, accounting for about 3,300 cases in 1998.)

Scientists often discuss the incidence of cancer in terms of rates. The incidence rate of colorectal cancer is the number of

---

* By "internal" I mean "other than skin cancers." Skin cancer is by far the most common form of cancer, accounting for more than 700,000 new cases each year. But the vast majority of skin cancers (95 percent) are superficial—and highly curable—forms of the disease.

new cases diagnosed in a particular year, divided by the population of the United States during that same year. The rates are often expressed as cases diagnosed per 100,000 people. The incidence rate of colorectal cancer is also decreasing; between 1990 and 1994, colorectal cancer incidence rates declined 7 percent, from 48 per 100,000 persons in 1990 to 44 per 100,000 persons in 1994.

The declining rate is a result of several factors. People have become more aware of the importance of maintaining a healthy lifestyle through eating a healthy diet, exercising, and seeing their doctors for regular checkups. What's more, as Louise discovered, advances in diagnosing colorectal cancer allow doctors to spot the problem earlier and to treat it, and even cure it, before it becomes a life-threatening illness. This positive progress underscores the message of this book: Thousands of cases of colorectal cancer—and thousands of deaths from the disease—can be prevented each year.

An exception to the overall decline is found among African American men. In this group, the incidence rate of colorectal cancer and the numbers of deaths from the disease are actually on the rise. For unknown reasons, colorectal cancer in African Americans tends to develop more often in the right (ascending) colon and is consequently harder to spot with routine screening.

Most people with colorectal cancer live with their disease for many years. Thus, another way to describe the impact of the disease is to cite its prevalence—the number of living people in whom a cancer has been diagnosed. The prevalence of colorectal cancer in this country is about 1,200,000 people. Approximately 840,000 of these cases involve colon cancer and 335,000 are rectal cancer.

Colorectal cancer can be fatal. Besides being the fourth most common cancer, it is second only to lung cancer as the leading cause of cancer-related deaths. Approximately 56,000 people will die this year because of the disease. Colorectal cancer accounts for roughly 3 percent of all deaths in the United States.

The overall five-year survival rate—the percentage of people who will live at least five years after their colorectal cancer is diagnosed—is about 61 percent. To be precise, the rate is about 62 percent for colon cancer and 60 percent for rectal cancer. Thanks to advances in diagnosis and treatment, the rate has improved dramatically since the early 1960s, when it was only 42 percent for colon cancer and 37 percent for rectal cancer.

The overall survival rate, however, is a somewhat confusing and misleading figure. There is nothing magical about the five-year benchmark. Many people live full and happy lives for much longer than five years after their diagnosis. Also, the survival rate reflects all reports of colorectal cancer, including the most severe cases. It does not indicate any differences in the survival rate based on the stage at diagnosis. If the cancer is detected in the earliest stages—before it has penetrated the surface of the intestine, and when a simple surgical procedure can result in a complete cure—the five-year survival rate is much higher: 92 percent for colon cancer and 85 percent for rectal cancer. These very positive numbers offer further proof of the importance of early detection.

OTHER FACTORS AFFECTING THE RATE OF COLORECTAL CANCER

Overall, the risk that a person will develop colorectal cancer at some point in his lifetime is about 1 in 17. Of the estimated 131,600 cases in 1998, roughly 64,600 will affect men and about 67,000 will develop in women.

Between the sexes, there is a minor difference in the part of the intestine where cancer develops. Among men, 69 percent of colorectal cancers develop in the colon. Among women, this figure is closer to 76 percent. According to some studies, women are more likely to develop anal cancers than men. However, homosexual men who engage in anal intercourse appear to be at higher risk of anal cancer than those who do not.

Age is a big factor in colorectal cancer. The longer you live, the greater your chances of developing the disease. Between 90 percent and 94 percent of cases are diagnosed in individuals who are fifty years of age or older. The risk continues to increase with age. The largest number of cases are diagnosed in people seventy-five years old. In contrast, anal cancer is more common among people between the ages of forty and sixty years.

The worldwide statistics tell an interesting story about the impact of culture on the incidence of colorectal cancer. The lowest rate occurs among people of India, where the disease affects only between 1 and 3 individuals per 100,000 population (roughly 1/20th the rate in the West). In westernized, industrialized nations, rates are approximately 25 to 35 cases per 100,000 people. The highest rates occur among white people (Caucasians) of northern European origin. The incidence is somewhat lower among white people of southern European heritage. Rates are lower among Asians, Native Americans, Pacific Islanders, and Hispanics than among whites. In Africa, the rate among blacks is much lower than among whites. In the United States, the rate among blacks is slightly higher than among whites.

By themselves, these numbers do not paint a complete picture. Studies of nonwhite people who migrate to Western countries show a dramatic increase, within just one or two generations, in the risk of colorectal cancer. In other words, within twenty to forty years after moving from India to Indiana, a person's risk of colorectal cancer increases by a factor of 20 until it equals the risk of people who have lived in the United States all their lives.

The conclusion from such studies is clear: Lifestyle, not ethnic origin, plays a critical role in the risk of colorectal cancer. Specifically, the typical Western diet—high in animal fat and low in fiber from fruits and vegetables—coupled with lack of exercise (plus various other factors) increases the risk.

Knowing that lifestyle is a risk factor allows us to take important steps toward preventing the disease. Keeping the disease from starting in the first place is known as primary prevention.

Screening—undergoing medical tests to look for colorectal cancer, even when no signs or symptoms are present—is another critical step. Treating noncancerous tumors to keep them from progressing to the point where they become cancerous is known as secondary prevention. Chapters 4 through 6 discuss these methods of prevention in more detail.

HOW IS COLORECTAL CANCER TREATED?

The "Resources" section at the end of the book describes some available methods for dealing with colorectal cancer. Here, too, the news is very good. Advances in the field in the past two decades have improved the outlook enormously. New technology lets us see polyps and tumors so we can treat them—and often cure them—at early stages in their development. (The process of obtaining an accurate diagnosis is covered in Chapter 7.)

As described in Chapter 8, modern surgical techniques allow physicians to remove affected areas of tissue with a low risk of long-term side effects. Apart from the fear of pain or an early death, the central concern for many people and their families as they cope with colorectal cancer is that the bowel will no longer function, requiring the use of an external bag to collect waste through a hole in the abdomen (colostomy). As I will explain, however, the risk of a permanent colostomy following surgical treatment is currently very low—around 3 percent.

For more advanced cases of colorectal cancer, radiation therapy and anticancer drugs can often add years to a person's life. Much of the improvement in the survival rates for colorectal cancer has resulted from the advances in these areas. Chapter 9 explains how these therapies work and what to expect from them.

In Chapter 10, I will discuss alternative or complementary therapies for colorectal cancer. Later chapters offer thoughts on how to deal with the health care system and emphasize the importance of follow-up care and of remaining vigilant against recurrence of the disease.

As a gastroenterologist who has specialized in colorectal cancer for more than twenty-five years, I am excited about the progress I have seen in this field, especially in the area of prevention. Each year, the United States Government invests millions of dollars in research on the disease. (Still, the money spent on research never seems to be enough, especially when this disease remains such a prevalent and deadly problem.) Genetic studies are leading to simple blood tests that will help us identify people who are at greatest risk. Scientists continue to discover new therapies and combinations of treatments that enable people to live fully active lives for many years.

By paying careful attention to diet, exercise, and other lifestyle factors, and by remaining vigilant for warning signs, it is possible to prevent colorectal cancer from developing in the first place. And prevention is the best treatment of all.

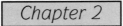

Inside the Body

This chapter explains the process of digestion and describes the organs involved. The main goal of this brief anatomy lesson is to make you familiar with the functions and the vocabulary associated with the parts of the body affected by colorectal cancer. If you or someone in your family is dealing with the disease, this information will help you realize what is happening internally. You will be better able to discuss your symptoms and reactions with your health care providers and to understand what happens during treatment.

Another goal of this chapter is to set the stage for later discussion of how a proper diet—low in animal fats; high in vegetables, fruits, and fiber—can go a long way toward preventing, or at least lowering the risk of, colorectal cancer.

The colon and the rectum represent the last phases of the digestive process. To understand what happens inside these organs, however, we need to start at the beginning.

DIGESTION

Digestion is the process of reducing food to small particles so that the body can absorb the nutrients—vitamins, minerals, and so on—that the food contains. The process of digestion actually begins as soon as food is put into the mouth. Chewing breaks the

Many people find it very difficult to talk about medical problems involving the digestive tract. In our society, such natural processes as excretion and elimination are either the subjects of off-color jokes, or they are taboo. Between these two extremes, it is no wonder that people find it extremely embarrassing or distasteful to discuss these processes, even with their physicians. Unfortunately, this reluctance causes qualms about discussing a problem openly and honestly.

Marian is a case in point. For several weeks, this 58-year-old fashion boutique owner had noticed blood in the toilet following her bowel movements, one of the warning signs of cancer. She felt shocked and horrified, but was afraid to call her doctor. Eventually, she confided the problem to a friend, who persuaded her to call an internist and ask for an appointment. When the receptionist asked Marian if she was having any specific problems, she said, "No, just a little upset stomach now and then."

During the exam, she again denied that anything was wrong, but did manage to mention that her stools seemed "a little, well, loose once in a while." The doctor said he would like to perform a digital rectal exam (DRE), a simple test during which he would insert a gloved, lubricated finger into her rectum to check for signs of trouble. Marian asked if it was really necessary, and the doctor assured her it was quick and painless. Still she hesitated, and wondered if she might be able to schedule the test for another time when she could be "more prepared."

Fortunately, Marian's doctor had a good bedside manner. He realized how difficult it was for this dignified woman to subject herself to such poking and prodding, let alone talk about any problem she might be having. But he also sensed that she was deeply worried about something. He patiently explained that many people felt exactly the way she did. The DRE might not be pleasant to think about, but it was an important aspect of her medical care. Somewhat reassured, Marian agreed to the procedure, which revealed the presence of fresh blood. The internist referred Marian to me, and I found that she had an early-stage—and very treatable—cancer in her rectum.

The lesson is clear. When it comes to dealing with colorectal cancer, silence is not golden. The subject may be hard to talk about, but it's better to overcome those fears than to die because of embarrassment.

food into smaller pieces. Saliva and enzymes in the mouth dissolve and break down the food even more.

Swallowed food travels down a tube (called the esophagus) that connects the throat to the stomach (Figure 2.1). Inside the stomach, gastric juice—a fluid mixture of acid, mucus, and enzymes—dissolves the food into a semiliquid paste known as chyme (pronounced "kyme"). The churning motion of the stomach muscles also helps the process of dissolving.

The length of time food remains in the stomach (and in other parts of the digestive tract) depends on its ingredients. Carbohydrates are digested fastest—within one or two hours. Fatty foods take longest—from three to six hours. Proteins fall somewhere in between. Some nutrients, such as salt and sugar, are absorbed in the stomach, but the real work of absorption is accomplished later by the small intestine.

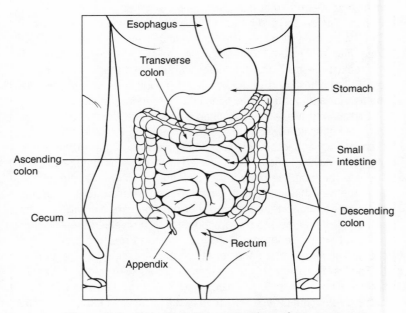

Figure 2.1: The digestive system's main organs.

Muscle contractions squeeze the digested material out of the stomach through a valve and into the small intestine. The word "small" refers to the organ's diameter—a little more than an inch—and not to its length, which is about eighteen to twenty-three feet.

The small intestine has three parts: (1) the duodenum, (2) the jejunum, and (3) the ileum. The duodenum is a C-shaped tube about ten inches long. Inside the duodenum, the chyme mixes with digestive secretions from two nearby organs, the pancreas and the gallbladder. The pancreas releases pancreatic juice, a fluid rich in enzymes (chemicals whose function is to split molecules of starch, protein, and fat into smaller pieces).

The gallbladder supplies bile, which is manufactured in the liver. Ingredients in bile, known as bile salts, help the body digest fats. Just as detergent breaks up oil, bile salts break fat globules into smaller droplets and help them mix with water. These smaller pieces can then be digested more easily by the action of pancreatic enzymes. Bile salts also help the intestine absorb fatty acids and vitamins that dissolve in fats, such as vitamins A, D, E, and K.

The more fat you eat, the more bile is released from the gallbladder. Most of the bile is absorbed by the small intestine. It then circulates, in the blood, back to the liver, which releases it again into the gallbladder where it is stored to await the next meal. Some bile remains in the chyme, however. Recent research suggests that the acids in bile may play a role in irritating cells in the large intestine, which in turn may contribute to the development of colorectal cancer.

The jejunum and the ileum make up most of the long, looping small intestine. These two parts have essentially the same functions: to continue digestion, absorb nutrients from the chyme, and keep the material churning and moving along through a series of rhythmic muscular contractions. Glands in the small intestine secrete a watery fluid filled with enzymes that break down molecules into smaller parts.

Inside the small intestine are thousands of tiny fingerlike projections called villi (plural of villus). They line the inside of the intestine like the fur lining of a glove. Each villus is covered with countless smaller projections called microvilli. These structures pick up the various molecules of water, fats, sugars, and proteins, and transport them into nearby small blood vessels. The nutrients then circulate throughout the body to the individual cells, which use them to carry out the various processes that keep the body alive.

Depending on the food consumed, it takes a meal between 20 minutes and 10 hours to make its way along the entire winding length of the small intestine. The process of digestion is very efficient. The small intestine absorbs most of the material, so that by the time it is ready to enter the large intestine only a relatively small amount remains.

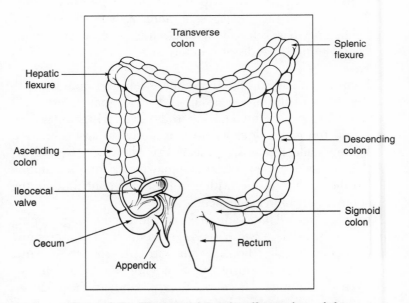

Figure 2.2: The large intestine (front view: right side of diagram is the left side of the body).

THE LARGE INTESTINE

The large intestine, or large bowel, is about five or six feet long and a little less than three inches in diameter (Figure 2.2). It begins on the lower right side of the body, rises up, crosses the abdomen, and descends on the left.

The outside layer of the intestine is called the serosa. Muscular strips running the length of this outer surface pull the organ into a series of pouches and give the colon its characteristic rippled look.

The spot where the small and large intestines join is guarded by the ileocecal valve. Normally, this muscular valve remains shut to prevent chyme from flowing backward from the large intestine. Impulses from elsewhere in the digestive tract—for example, signals from the stomach indicating another meal is being eaten—trigger muscle contractions that force digested material through the valve and into the first chamber of the intestine, known as the cecum. Dangling below the cecum is a narrow tube called the appendix. (Why we have an appendix is a mystery. It does not contribute anything to the digestive process, although it may help in the fight against infection.)

The main function of the colon is to absorb moisture from the chyme. As the material moves along, it becomes drier and firmer.

The colon has four parts; their names reflect the direction in which the chyme moves (Figure 2.3). The ascending (or right) colon begins at the cecum and rises upward. Digested material—at this point, still mainly fluid—may stay in the ascending colon for up to twenty-four hours.

At the end of the ascending section, the colon takes a sharp left turn. Here it becomes the transverse colon, so called because it crosses (transverses) the abdomen. The transverse colon, the longest section of the organ, is held in place by a fatty, apronlike membrane called the omentum. The transverse colon does not run straight across the abdomen. Instead, it sags in the middle.

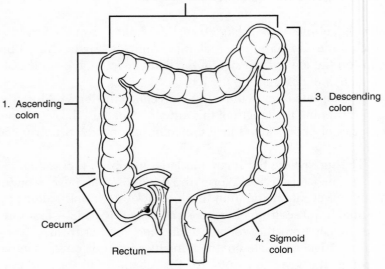

Figure 2.3: The four parts of the colon. The cecum is the connection to the small intestine. The rectum is a conduit to the anal canal.

On the left side of the body, the intestine takes another ninety-degree turn where the descending (or left) colon begins. At a point roughly aligned with the cecum on the opposite side, the colon turns back to the right and begins to form an S-shape, not unlike the trap in the drain underneath a sink. This section is named the sigmoid colon (after sigma, the S-shaped letter of the Greek alphabet). The viewing tool doctors use to examine this lower portion of the colon is called a sigmoidoscope.

Knowing the sections of the intestine can help with understanding more about the nature of colorectal cancer. For one thing, tumors developing in different areas may cause distinctive patterns of symptoms. Cancer in the descending colon, for example, is more likely to cause intestinal blockage than cancer in the ascending portion — in part, because the feces at this point contain less water and are more solid. In contrast, weakness due to loss of blood (anemia) is often a symptom of cancer in the right colon but is infrequent when cancer occurs in the left colon. The location of a tumor determines how it will be treated.

At the end of the sigmoid colon is the rectum, which is about six to eight inches long. This muscular chamber serves primarily as a container for feces just before excretion. (The word feces is plural and it comes from the Latin word for "dregs.") Pressure caused by feces moving into the rectum triggers the sensation of needing to go to the bathroom. Attached to the rectum is the anal canal, a short channel about two or three inches long. This ends in the anus, the muscular opening through which feces are eliminated during defecation.

By the time chyme enters the large intestine from the small intestine, most of the work of digestion has been completed. There are no villi inside the large intestine, so not much absorption takes place there, although the colon does absorb water and electrolytes (such as sodium and potassium). As the remaining material moves through the colon, it gradually becomes a semisolid mass consisting of indigestible food such as fiber, sloughed-off cells from the lining of the digestive tract, water, mucus, and various other substances. About half the weight of the feces is dead bacteria from the large intestine. Bile gives the material its brown color. The odor results from substances such as sulfide and ammonia that are produced by bacterial activity.

A CLOSER LOOK

Other parts of the large intestine are worth discussing because they play a role in colorectal cancer. The basic fact to keep in mind here is that cancer starts when something causes the cells on the inner lining of the intestine to mutate and grow out of control. As these growths progress, they affect deeper and deeper layers of cells. If they are not treated in time, these growths can become cancerous. They can damage the intestine, penetrate from the inner surface to the outer surface of the intestine, and spread to other parts of the body. The next chapter describes that progression more fully.

A cross section of the colon wall reveals that it is made up of several distinct layers, like the rings that are visible in a slice taken from a tree trunk (Figure 2.4). There are four main rings. The innermost ring of the colon is known as the mucous membrane (or the **mucosa**). The topmost layer of the mucosa, the epithelium, contains cells that line the colon. These cells form columns with spaces, or crypts, between them. Most colorectal cancers begin as microscopic changes in the cells found along these crypts. (You will learn more about these cells in the following chapter, which discusses the origin and progression of cancer in greater detail.) The cells of the epithelium are supported by a thin layer called the

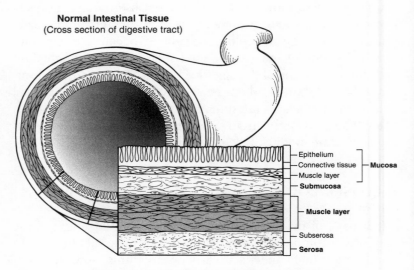

Figure 2.4: The layers of the colon wall.

basement membrane. Beneath that is a layer of connective tissue (the lamina propria) and, finally, a thin layer of musclelike tissue (muscularis mucosae). This mucous membrane contains glands (mucosal glands), formed by cells, that secrete the fluid that makes up mucus. Mucus protects cells from damage and contributes lubricating moisture to the fecal material as it moves through the intestine.

The next major "ring" is the submucosa, a layer that contains connective tissue, blood vessels, lymphatic vessels, and nerves.

Then there is a layer of muscular tissue. These muscles contract and expand to help move the feces along toward the rectum.

The outermost layer—the "bark" of the colon, to continue the image of the tree rings—is called the serosa. Between the serosa and the muscle layer is a band of connective tissue referred to as the subserosa.

This microscopic look at the colon is offered to help you understand the concept of cancer staging. Abnormal growths on the surface (epithelium) of the mucosa are relatively easy to see during an endoscopic examination. Just as important, these superficial growths can be easily removed through a simple surgical procedure. This step prevents cancer from developing, or it results in a complete cure if cancer has begun. However, once the growth penetrates any of the deeper layers of the colon or rectum, including the muscle layer or the serosa, the problem becomes much more serious and the outlook is less hopeful.

As is the case everywhere in the body, the tissues in the colon and rectum are fed by networks of blood vessels and nerves. Another network that is of tremendous importance in any discussion of cancer is the lymphatic system. This system, which basically parallels the bloodstream, performs many essential functions. In a sense, the lymphatic system serves as the body's water purification plant. It absorbs fluid that leaks out of blood capillaries and cells during normal metabolism and returns it to the bloodstream. This whitish or yellowish fluid, called lymph, contains cells, dead bacteria, and other particles that result when the body fights off infection. Lymph circulates in vessels to the lymph nodes. These nodes work as filters to trap the particles and remove them from the fluid before it returns to the bloodstream.

Unfortunately, the lymphatic system also plays a role in the spread of cancer. Cancerous cells that break off from a tumor can get picked up in the lymph fluid, which then transports them to other tissues. During surgery to remove a tumor, surgeons will usually take out a number of neighboring lymph nodes. A pathologist studies the nodes to determine the presence of any cancer cells. The more nodes that contain cancer cells, the more advanced—and the more dangerous—the cancer. The concept of cancer staging, described in more detail in the following chapter, is a system for describing how far the cancer has spread within the body.

SUMMARY

The key points in this chapter are:

- Colorectal cancer develops in the last part of the digestive tract.
- Substances contained in the digested material can irritate cells that line the inner surface of the intestine.
- Changes in these cells can lead to the development of abnormal growths, which, over time, can become cancerous.

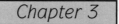

How Cancer Develops

Cancer is a disease that causes cells to grow in an abnormal and dangerous way. To understand how colorectal cancer develops, how it affects the body, and how treatment works, it helps to be familiar with what cells do.

The human body is made up of billions of cells. These tiny structures are responsible for carrying out the basic activities of life. Cells are like factories. They take in raw materials (nutrients) that have been absorbed from food, and they use them to assemble complex molecules called proteins. Proteins form the basis for tissues and organs. They are also the key ingredient in hormones, enzymes, antibodies, and many other substances in the body.

There are many different types of cells in the body. Most of them perform the same basic functions, but each type also specializes in carrying out one or more different tasks. Cells in endocrine glands, for example, secrete hormones; muscle cells contract to move different parts of the body; and nerve cells carry electrical signals from the brain.

Cells in some organs constantly reproduce themselves. Reproduction is necessary because certain types of cells live for only a limited amount of time. The cells in the lining of the large intestine, for example, die after four to six days. New cells must constantly take the place of the old ones. Cells multiply by dividing. Normal cells live, divide, and die in a fixed pattern and at a fixed rate.

Each new "daughter" cell must be an exact copy of its parent if it is to function properly. To understand this process, it is necessary to take a closer look inside the cell.

DNA'S ROLE

The cell's instructions for making proteins are contained in molecules called DNA (a short name for *d*eoxyribo-*n*ucleic *a*cid). These molecules, housed in the cell's central unit (the nucleus), are shaped like long twisted ladders (Figure 3.1). Each "rung" of the ladder is made of two different molecules (called bases) that are attached in the center. There are only four kinds of base molecules in DNA: (1) adenine, (2) cytosine, (3) guanine, and (4) thymine. They are identified in short

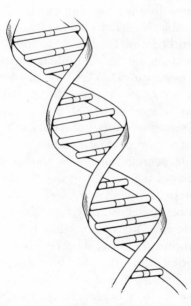

Figure 3.1: The ladder shape of DNA molecules.

form, as A, C, G, and T. Each base can only be paired with a certain mate: A can only attach to T, and C can only attach to G. These base pairs are like an alphabet of life. Segments of DNA, known as genes, contain a precise sequence of the pairs. Just as the order of letters determines the meaning of a word, the sequences of the "rungs" determine what protein a gene will produce. If there is a flaw in the gene—if a rung is missing, or if it is made with a wrong base molecule—the cell will produce faulty proteins.

When a cell reproduces, the DNA inside the nucleus splits down the middle, as if the rungs of the ladder were being sawed in half. (For this discussion, think of these two sections as the left and the right halves.) Base molecules floating around in the cell then attach themselves to their "mates" on the half-rungs. For example, a new C molecule will be drawn to the G on the left half of the ladder. Meanwhile, a new G will be drawn to the C on the right half. When each base molecule has attracted its specific mate, the result is two complete and exact copies of the original DNA molecule. Once that process is complete, a new functioning cell has been born.

Every day, millions of our cells divide and reproduce in the normal, healthy way. But just as a "bug" in a software program can cause a computer to crash, something can happen to the cell that disrupts its normal life cycle. To put it simply, these disruptions sometimes result in the disease we call cancer.

For example, some of the instructions contained in DNA tell the cell when it is time to reproduce, and others determine when it is time to die. This is known as programmed cell death (or, in the scientific jargon, apoptosis). Cell death is an important aspect of any discussion of cancer. If the cell lacks this particular set of instructions, or if the gene that regulates apoptosis is missing or becomes damaged, the cell may reproduce many times, at a rapid rate, without dying. These damaged cells crowd out healthy cells and eventually produce a mass called a tumor. In other cases, the defect may cause the cell to cease making proteins, or to make faulty proteins that fail to carry out their function inside the body. Some cells become so defective that they damage their neighbors, penetrate other nearby tissues, and enter the bloodstream or lymphatic system. If that happens, they can travel to other locations in the body, start new tumors, and cause widespread damage.

The body contains many types of cells, and each type has a specific function. Cancer can affect just about any of these various cells. For that reason, it helps to think of cancer not as a single disease but as many diseases. There are more than a hundred kinds of cancers, each with its own characteristics, treatments, and outcomes. It is important to bear this in mind, because cancer affects different people in dramatically different ways. If you are dealing with colorectal cancer, resist the temptation to compare your situation to that of a relative or friend who also has the disease or who has cancer in another part of the body. No two cases are exactly alike.

The cell defects that result in cancer can occur in several ways. A foreign or harmful substance may penetrate the cell and its nucleus, damaging one or more vital parts of the DNA. Environmental factors—cancer-causing factors found in the world around us—include the quality of the air we breathe and the water we drink, as well as basic lifestyle choices such as diet, use of alcohol and tobacco, and the amount of exercise we get.

A person's DNA may have been faulty to begin with. This is what we mean when we talk about *hereditary* genetic defects. Any flaws in the DNA found in a father's sperm or a mother's egg will be recreated every time a cell divides in the developing fetus. Some time later in life, something may happen to cause that defect to manifest itself. I will discuss the hereditary forms of colorectal cancer a little later in this chapter.

The basic point to remember is that cancer is a disease in which cells become abnormal: they multiply without control and crowd out healthy cells. What causes the abnormality to occur and result in colorectal cancer is not always clear. As I will explain in a moment, many cases probably result from some combination of environmental and hereditary factors. The more we understand about these factors, the greater is the chance that we can prevent colorectal cancer.

SOME IMPORTANT CONCEPTS IN COLORECTAL CANCER

Cancer is a confusing, complex illness. In this section, I will define a few of the important terms that will come up often in any discussion of the disease. The more informed you are about the nature of the disease, the easier it will be for you to understand how to prevent it, or how to deal with doctors and treatments if the disease occurs.

When cells grow out of control, they collect and form into a mass called a tumor. The word tumor comes from the Latin term for a swelling. Some tumors are not dangerous to health or life. The cells merely accumulate in one place. The swelling may produce discomfort, pain, bleeding, or other unpleasant symptoms, but the cells do not penetrate or damage nearby tissues, nor do they migrate to other locations in the body. Such tumors are not cancerous or life-threatening. We refer to them as *benign* tumors. A common example of a benign tumor, familiar to most women, is a fibroid tumor, which typically develops in the uterus.

Tumors that invade neighboring tissues and organs or migrate (metastasize) to other sites are cancerous. These are called *malignant* tumors, also known as cancer. Cancers that attack other parts of the body powerfully or quickly are often referred to as aggressive cancers.

Inside the colon and rectum, something can happen to accelerate the growth of certain cells. Over time, a benign tumor known as a polyp can develop.

As I explained in Chapter 1, polyps start off as harmless, but, over time, they can become cancerous. This process, known as *progression*, is important in a discussion of colorectal cancer prevention. If polyps are detected early through careful screening and diagnosis, they can be easily and completely removed in a minor procedure called a *polypectomy*. Removing the polyp ends its chances of turning into cancer. We'll take a closer look at how polyps progress into malignant tumors a bit later.

The term *primary cancer* refers to the site of the first tumor. A diagnosis of "primary colorectal cancer" indicates that the disease first developed inside the colon or rectum. Cancer cells that metastasize to another part of the body can start new tumors. If colorectal cancer spreads, the cells typically travel, first, to the lymph nodes and then to the liver, lungs, or abdominal (peritoneal) cavity. Tumors that result from metastasis are called *secondary cancer* or *metastatic cancer*. Colorectal cancer that has traveled to the liver, for example, is diagnosed not as liver cancer but as metastatic (or secondary) colorectal cancer. (Tumors that develop first in the liver would be diagnosed as primary liver cancer.)

For most purposes, the terms "spread" and "metastasis" can be used interchangeably without confusion. In precise usage, however, *spread* refers to cancerous cells that invade tissues or organs immediately next to the original tumor. *Metastasis*, in contrast, refers to cells that break off from the tumor and travel away from the original site.

Recurrent cancer describes a tumor that returns after treatment, either at the original (primary) site or at another location. The rate of recurrence of primary colorectal cancer is relatively high: between 30 percent and 40 percent of people who undergo surgery to cure colorectal cancer are likely to experience a return of the disease.

SYMPTOMS OF COLORECTAL CANCER

It is important to understand that some cases of colorectal cancer cause no symptoms whatsoever, especially in the early stages.

Polyps may grow inside the intestine and, over time, may transform into cancer without sending out any signals that something's wrong. By the time symptoms do develop, the cancer may have metastasized, at which point a surgical cure is not possible. This is why screening for the disease—looking for signs of trouble even though everything appears normal—is essential for preventing it. (For more information about screening, see Chapter 6.)

In more advanced cases, however, colorectal cancer can cause symptoms (see box). The first warning sign is often a change in the normal pattern of bowel movements. Some people may have fewer movements than normal; others may have movements more frequently. Keep in mind that what is "normal" varies from person to person. For some people, regular movements might mean once a day; for others, every two or three days or two or three times each

---

Possible Symptoms of Colorectal Cancer
- Change in bowel habits
  —Diarrhea
  —Constipation
  —Narrow stools
- Blood in the stool
- Weakness or fatigue (as a result of anemia from loss of blood)
- Cramping or gnawing abdominal pain
- Loss of appetite or nausea
- Weight loss
- Straining during a bowel movement (more common with rectal cancer)

Possible Symptoms of Anal Cancer
- Bleeding from the anus (even a small amount)
- Pain or pressure in the area around the anus
- Itching or discharge
- Lump in the anal area
- Straining during a bowel movement

day might be normal. The point is that colorectal cancer can cause a *change* in the normal pattern. Some people experience difficulty passing stools (constipation); others have frequent, loose, or watery stools (diarrhea). Often, the symptom involves a narrowing in the diameter of the feces. This can result if a tumor is present and is reducing the width of the intestine.

Blood in the stool is another common symptom. The blood may appear in the toilet bowl following the bowel movement, or it may appear as streaks in the feces. Sometimes the blood appears on toilet tissue after wiping, or it may stain bedsheets or undergarments. Be aware, however, that blood in feces may not be visible. Doctors can perform a simple test on a stool sample to detect the presence of hidden (occult) blood. (For more information, see Chapter 6.)

If bleeding is severe, it may lead to iron-deficiency anemia, which causes a general feeling of weakness or fatigue. Iron is necessary in the blood because it helps to carry to the cells the oxygen they need to burn calories and convert food to energy.

Other possible symptoms of colorectal cancer include recurring discomfort, cramps, or pain in the abdominal area. Some people experience constant nausea (queasy stomach). Not surprisingly, problems involving digestion can often take away one's appetite. Over time, the presence of colorectal cancer and its impact on the body, especially on the digestive system, can lead to a noticeable loss of weight.

If symptoms are present, their pattern may provide clues about the location of a tumor. (For more information on the various parts of the colon, see Chapter 2.) Cancer on the right (ascending) colon is more likely to involve rectal bleeding, anemia, and discomfort on the right side of the abdomen. About 25 percent of colorectal cancers develop in this region.

Tumors on the left (descending) or sigmoid colon tend to grow in a ring that completely encompasses the diameter of the organ. These tumors typically cause changes of bowel habits, obstruction (blocked passage of feces), and streaks of blood in the stool.

Blockage can lead to abdominal cramping and pain. Large tumors that almost completely block the intestine can lead to diarrhea. About 10 percent of tumors grow in the transverse colon (the horizontal segment that crosses the abdomen), 15 percent develop in the descending colon, and 20 percent are found in the sigmoid colon.

If a tumor is located in the rectum, a common sign is blood in the toilet bowl following a bowel movement. Tumors in the lower part of the rectum or in the anus may cause a sensation of pressure on tissues in the region. This pressure often leads to severe straining (what doctors call tenesmus) during a bowel movement. Roughly 30 percent of colorectal cancers develop in the rectum, while a small percentage (1 to 2 percent) affect the anus.

These signs and symptoms are not unique to colorectal cancer. They can be caused by any number of other diseases and medical conditions. To give a simple example, hemorrhoids—swellings that develop in the blood vessels surrounding the anus—can sometimes burst, resulting in rectal bleeding. If you or members of your family experience bleeding or abdominal pain, it is imperative that you seek medical evaluation. A doctor can conduct tests to pin down the cause of the problem.

FACTORS THAT MAY CAUSE—OR PROTECT AGAINST—COLORECTAL CANCER

It is difficult to state with certainty what causes precancerous polyps to develop in the colon and rectum, or what triggers their progression into cancer. Many different factors all come into play. As noted earlier, some of these are environmental and some are hereditary.

Keep in mind, too, that a "risk factor" is not the same as a cause. Colorectal cancer may never develop in someone who has several risk factors—such as a high-fat, low-fiber diet and a family history of the disease—but it might develop in someone who appears to have no risk factors.

Diet

Diets containing high levels of meat, protein, and animal fat are clearly associated with an increased risk of cancer in either the colon or the rectum. The risk appears to be higher (especially for rectal cancer) if the meat is routinely fried, or cooked at high temperatures until it is well done, but some people may have inherited a genetic trait that keeps their bodies from absorbing certain substances found in heavily cooked meat that are suspected of causing cancer.

Many scientific studies have shown quite conclusively that when the amount of fiber in the diet goes up, the risk of colorectal cancer goes down. Of the several types of fiber, the kind that appears to be especially protective comes from vegetables, but fruits and grains also contribute helpful types of fiber. Foods rich in calcium, vitamin C, or a B vitamin called folate may also have a protective effect. People who eat large amounts of fish or seafood also appear to be at less risk.

Eating fat triggers the release of bile, and bile acids are suspected as a cause of colorectal cancer. A handful of studies have reported that eating frequent meals, especially meals with a high fat content, might raise the risk to some degree. The following chapter offers more suggestions for choosing a diet to lower the risk of colorectal cancer.

Alcohol

There is some evidence that drinking one to two alcoholic beverages each day may increase the risk of colorectal cancer, especially cancer of the rectum. The risk is slightly higher among men and among beer drinkers. Not all studies have found a relationship between alcohol consumption and risk of cancer, but none of the research suggests that alcohol actually protects against the disease. Alcohol may possibly stimulate cells in the intestine to reproduce more rapidly, or, if any cancer-causing substances are already present, alcohol may accelerate the damage they cause to the cells.

Smoking

Use of tobacco is clearly related to cancer in the lung and other parts of the body. Recent studies have found evidence that habitual smokers, particularly those who have smoked for thirty-five years or longer, may be at high risk of colorectal cancer, especially for tumors developing in the rectum. Some researchers note that pipes or cigars may present more risk than cigarettes, possibly because cancer-causing chemicals from these forms of tobacco usage are more likely to be swallowed. The longer people use these products, and the earlier in life they begin smoking, the higher their chance of developing colorectal cancer later in life.

Cigarette smoking appears to increase the risk of precancerous polyps, and smokers run a higher risk than nonsmokers of having polyps grow back after they have been removed. This is important because although polyps begin as benign growths, they can turn into cancerous tumors. According to one study, perhaps 20 percent of large-bowel cancers in men may have originated as smoking-induced polyps.

Physical Exercise

Studies consistently find that people who do not get enough exercise are at higher risk of colorectal cancer. People who have active jobs or who take part in leisure-time sports have lower rates of the disease, especially if they have been active all their lives (as opposed to having started an exercise regimen later in life).

Weight

Obesity (being more than 20 percent over average body weight for one's height) may increase the risk of colorectal cancer. Overweight people have an *energy imbalance:* they generally consume more calories than they expend during the day. Excess calories may speed up the rate at which the body's cells reproduce. Or, restricting calories and reducing body mass may protect against cancer by slowing down the rate of cell growth or interfering with some other step in the process by which benign tumors progress to cancerous ones.

Reproductive Status

Intriguingly, nuns—a population of women who do not bear children and who do not need to take hormones for birth control—have higher rates of several forms of cancer, including colorectal cancer. This has led researchers to examine whether female hormones offer any protective benefits. The evidence is not very strong, but it appears that the more children a woman has (and thus, the more hormones her body produces), the lower her risk of colorectal cancer. Similarly, while use of estrogen to relieve symptoms of menopause may increase the risk of liver or breast cancer, it does not increase—and may even lower—the risk of colorectal cancer. More studies are needed, however, before we can state any certain relationship between female hormones and colorectal cancer risk.

Occupation

People who work in certain jobs may be at higher risk of colorectal cancer, especially cancer of the rectum. Some (but not all) studies have found that rates of colorectal cancer tend to be higher among painters, printers, railway workers, woodworkers, automobile workers, and those who handle substances such as pesticides and herbicides. According to some reports, people who are heavily exposed to asbestos, a fiberlike mineral once used in insulation, develop colorectal cancer at twice the normal rate.

Making Sense of the Science

To summarize:

- The risk of colorectal cancer is higher among people whose diets are high in meat, fat, and protein, especially if those diets are also low in fiber from vegetables and fruits.
- Cooking meats at high temperatures may cause normally harmless substances to change into cancer-causing carcinogens—the same type of harmful substances found in tobacco. Some people are born with an inability to metabolize these substances effectively, which may make them more susceptible to cancer from these sources.
- The body releases bile to digest fatty foods. The longer cells in the bowel are exposed to bile acids, the greater the chance that they can be damaged. However, fiber appears to "attach" itself to bile acids, helping these molecules to pass through the bowel more quickly and thus reducing the risk of damage to the cells.
- Foods contain many different kinds of nutrients, and we do not yet know precisely which nutrients help prevent cancer and which ones may promote it. Eating a balanced diet that includes a variety of foods is the most sensible strategy.
- Lack of exercise can reduce the speed with which the intestine processes and eliminates food—a negative effect.
- Overeating can lead to being overweight, which can result in hormonal changes, lack of exercise, and an energy imbalance. All of these may increase the risk of cancer.
- Some people inherit damaged genes that make them more susceptible to developing polyps, which, over time, can become cancerous.

HEREDITY

Some forms of cancer tend to run in families. Hereditary factors may be involved to some extent in as many as 10 to 20 percent of colorectal cancers. (Cases that are not hereditary are known as sporadic cancers.)

People who have a first-degree relative (parent or sibling) with colorectal cancer are at double or triple the risk of getting the disease themselves. Some evidence also suggests that a family history of cancer in other organs (such as the breasts or ovaries) increases the risk that first-degree relatives will develop colorectal cancer. When discussing family risk, it can be hard to separate factors due to heredity from factors due to the environment, because family members living in the same home usually eat the same types of food and lead similar lifestyles. Further evidence of a genetic link comes from studies showing that second- and third-degree relatives (such as cousins) of people with a particular form of hereditary colorectal cancer are at a higher risk of getting the disease than the average population. Such findings argue for a genetic link to colorectal cancer, because these relatives usually do not share the same environment, the way first-degree relatives do.

As noted in Chapter 1, two major inherited conditions lead directly to an increased risk of colorectal cancer: (1) familial adenomatous polyposis (FAP), which causes about 1 percent of colorectal cancer cases annually in the United States, and (2) hereditary nonpolyposis colorectal cancer (HNPCC), which causes between 1 and 5 percent of cases annually.

Let's discuss FAP first; we'll start by defining some important terms.

The word *familial* indicates that this is a condition that runs in a family. *Polyposis* means "a disease that causes growth of polyps." There are several kinds of polyps. Those that arise due to inflammation (inflammatory polyps) or that are caused by excessive, yet limited, cell growth (hyperplastic polyps) will not develop into cancer. Despite the sound of their name, hyperplastic polyps are not dangerous.

An adenomatous polyp (or adenoma) is a growth that develops in glandular tissue, such as the mucous membrane inside the large intestine. (The term *adeno-* means "gland.") Adenomatous polyps are not dangerous by themselves, but, in time, a small minority of these polyps can develop into malignant (cancerous) tumors. These polyps—sometimes referred to as precancerous growths—are a source of worry in people who have FAP.

As humans get older, and especially as they pass the age of sixty, there is a greater chance that a few polyps will grow inside the colon or rectum. As I've stated, some of these polyps may become cancerous. By comparison, people with FAP often have hundreds or even thousands of polyps in their large intestine. The polyps begin to grow quickly around the age of puberty and, in most cases, are clearly visible through a sigmoidoscope by the age of fifteen or sixteen years. The chance that at least some of these polyps will become cancerous—and potentially fatal—is very high; nearly 100 percent of people with FAP will develop colorectal cancer at some time in their lives. Colon cancer develops by age twenty-one in about 7 percent of people with FAP, and by age forty-five in 90 percent. For this reason, by the age of eighteen or so, people with FAP should consider having surgery to remove most or all of their colon and rectum before the cancer can develop. Taking this step can prevent cancer and add decades to their lives.

One form of FAP is a rare disease known as Gardner's syndrome, named after Eldon Gardner, the scientist who first described it. This inherited condition, which also involves the growth of hundreds of polyps in the colon, produces a number of other problems, including tumors or cysts on the skull bones (osteomas), skin, and other soft tissues. The treatment is the same: partial or complete surgical removal of the large intestine.

People who have the other genetic form of large-bowel cancer, HNPCC, do not produce the large numbers of polyps in the colon that are common in people with FAP. Instead, they usually have one or a few adenomatous polyps. However, these polyps tend to be large in size, and they develop at a younger age than in the general population.

HNPCC comes in two forms; both are named after Henry Lynch, the doctor who discovered them. Lynch syndrome I involves only colorectal cancer. Lynch syndrome II, sometimes called family cancer syndrome, is a condition in which members tend to have a higher incidence of other types of cancer, especially cancer of the lining of the uterus (endometrial cancer).

For a diagnosis of HNPCC to be made, the person with the disease must have at least two first-degree relatives who also have colorectal cancer, one of whom must belong to a different generation. At least one of these cases must involve a person fifty years of age or younger.

Generally, the outlook for people with HNPCC is better than for those with FAP. The average age at which colorectal cancer develops in the HNPCC population is forty-five years. People with this form of inherited risk should undergo colon examinations (colonoscopies) every one or two years beginning between the ages of twenty and thirty, and then annually after the age of forty. Once cancer develops, part or all of the intestine is usually surgically removed.

In the past few years, scientists working to uncover the genetic defects that cause these hereditary forms of colorectal cancer have identified a number of abnormal (mutant) genes, and a blood test is now available to identify people who have these conditions. From a medical perspective, the test makes it easier to screen for the disease, to monitor affected individuals, and to perform surgery that will prevent cancer from cutting their lives short. However, people who are considering genetic testing should first seek genetic counseling, to understand the potential disadvantages of a positive test result. They may be unable to obtain health insurance or to pay the high cost of that insurance. A doctor or genetic counselor can provide up-to-date information and help in weighing the pros and cons of genetic testing.

People who know they have a hereditary risk of colorectal cancer may be able to reduce the chance that the disease will occur, or at least delay its development, through the use of certain chemicals or other substances. This concept, known as chemoprevention, is discussed in Chapter 5.

OTHER DISEASES ASSOCIATED WITH COLORECTAL CANCER

People who have chronic inflammatory bowel diseases are at high risk of developing colorectal cancer. The two main culprits in this category are ulcerative colitis and Crohn's disease.

Ulcerative colitis is a disease in which the colon and rectum suffer repeated, prolonged episodes of inflammation. The inflamed tissue becomes irritated and red. Cells are unable to function properly. In time, open sores (ulcers) develop in the lining of the colon and rectum. The main symptoms include bloody diarrhea and feces that contain mucus and pus. In severe cases, abdominal pain and tenderness may be present, along with flulike symptoms (fever, aches, chills, and general weakness and weight loss). Bouts of symptoms may occur every few months, or they may be constant.

Crohn's disease can affect either the small intestine or the large intestine, or both. This condition is sometimes called regional enteritis, because it can affect some regions of the bowel while leaving other sections alone. Symptoms resemble those of ulcerative colitis: frequent attacks of diarrhea, abdominal pain, and flulike symptoms.

Because these chronic conditions can damage the cells that line the colon and rectum, they make colorectal cancer more likely to develop. The longer the disease is present, the greater the risk of colorectal cancer. People who have severe inflammatory bowel disease that has lasted at least eight to ten years are at highest risk. Those with chronic ulcerative colitis are at more risk than those with Crohn's disease. However, people in whom the disease affects only the left (descending) colon seem to be at a lower risk of cancer than those in whom the disease affects the entire bowel. We do not yet know what factors can lead to cancer in people with chronic inflammatory bowel disease, but it appears that a diet lacking in folate, a B vitamin, may be involved. Scientists are also trying to determine whether gene defects may play a role.

As with other forms of colorectal cancer, a diagnosis can be made by taking a tissue sample (biopsy) during a colonoscopy. This procedure should be done every year or two after the inflammatory disease has been present for at least eight years. The goal, again, is to detect abnormal growth patterns or abnormal cells before they become cancerous or, if that is not possible, to detect the presence of cancer before it spreads beyond the lining of the intestine.

CAUSES OF AND RISK FACTORS FOR ANAL CANCER

Cancer affecting the anus is of a different nature than cancer involving the colon or the rectum. Perhaps three out of four cases of anal cancer that invades surrounding tissue result from infection with human papilloma virus (HPV). There are several types of HPV; some cause relatively minor problems, such as warts and benign tumors (papillomas). However, some of the types of HPV that are transmitted through sexual activity, including anal intercourse, can cause more serious types of abnormal growths. As is the case with polyps, the warts produced by these high-risk forms of HPV can, in time, turn into cancer. Detecting and removing the growths through surgery can prevent anal cancer. In some cases, though, no warts are visible.

Cigarette smoking also appears to increase the risk of developing anal cancer.

THE DEVELOPMENT OF COLORECTAL CANCER

Cancers in the colon and rectum develop slowly, over a period of many years. The disease usually begins as noncancerous polyps. Then something happens to cause the benign polyps (adenomas) to transform into malignant tumors (carcinomas).

This process—called progression, conversion, or the adenoma–carcinoma sequence—is a blessing in disguise. Because it takes so long and occurs in distinct stages, it allows time to detect the growths and remove them before they can cause trouble. Its slow progression makes colorectal cancer a very preventable form of the disease.

It's worthwhile to devote some space to a discussion of this process and the terms involved. Knowledge of this specialized language will help you make sense of what your doctors tell you during screening for or diagnosis of colorectal cancer. You'll also have a realistic concept of colorectal cancer staging and how the stage of a tumor affects its treatment. I'll cover likely outcomes in the last part of this chapter.

THE PROCESS OF PROGRESSION

The adenoma–carcinoma sequence begins with normal cells in the colon or rectum. These cells lie inside tiny pockets, called *crypts*, in the surface of the mucous membrane that lines the intestine (Figure 3.2). Then an event occurs that disrupts the way the normal cells behave. The trigger might be a genetic problem

Crypts

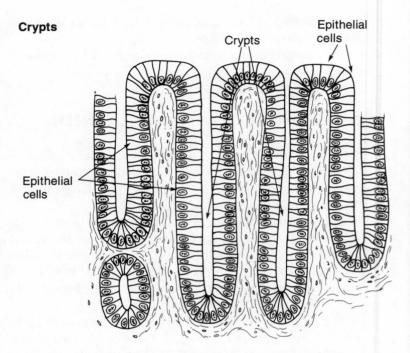

Figure 3.2: Cross section of the mucous membrane, showing the crypts, or spaces in the lining.

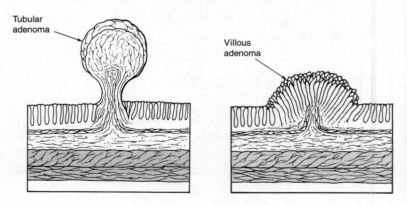

Figure 3.3: Polyps.

that suddenly kicks in, or the presence of a cancer-causing parti-cle in food that is being digested, or inflammation from a chronic bowel disease, or something else. Whatever the cause, the result is the same: the abnormal cells begin to multiply out of control, interfering with the activity of normal cells and refusing to die when their active time span should have ended.

In the very earliest phases, the cell defect may be too small to see with the naked eye. Under a microscope, however, a tiny crypt in the intestinal lining will appear abnormal—different from its many neighbors. The abnormal crypt has a larger diam-eter and a thicker layer of cells. The shape of the goblet cells—specialized cells that produce mucus—has become distorted. The technical term for these changes is *dysplasia*, which means "abnormal growth." A general term for such a change in tissue is a *lesion*.

In normal crypts, new cells are usually born at the bottom of the pocket. In abnormal crypts, the new cells may be produced closer to the surface of the mucous membrane. After a while, so many new cells grow that the lesion starts to bulge above the sur-face. This bulge or growth is called a polyp. As noted earlier, most polyps are harmless hyperplastic polyps.

Polyps that are at risk of becoming malignant are called adeno-mas or adenomatous polyps. Some may grow quite large; some be-come the size of an apple. Adenomatous polyps appear in several forms (Figure 3.3). Those with tube-shaped glands that end on the polyp's surface are called tubular adenomas. Those with sur-faces that look like bristles on a brush are called villous adenomas (villous means "shaped like villi," or fine hairs). Polyps that com-bine both features are known as tubulovillous adenomas. Polyps with a villous surface are more dangerous than tubular polyps, be-cause they have a greater risk of progressing to cancer.

Many polyps resemble mushrooms because they have a slender stalk below a kind of cap. Doctors call these polyps *pedunculated*. (*Ped-* means "foot" or "standing"; we get words such as "pedestal" from that root.)

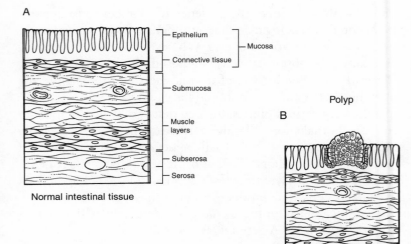

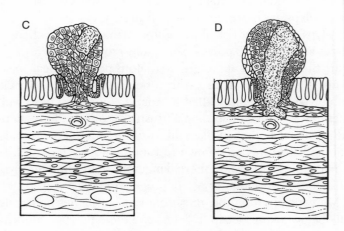

Figure 3.4: Cancer invading tissue.

Some polyps do not have a stalk (Figure 3.4B). These polyps are classified as *sessile* (from the Latin word for "sitting"). Sessile polyps are dangerous because they are likely to become cancerous. Some sessile lesions may be flat or indented (depressed). Over time, some of the polyps continue to change. Eventually, a certain percentage of them may start to form tumors that invade or grow into the connective tissue of the polyp stalk (Figure 3.4C) or into the tissue of the adjacent normal area of the colon or rectum (Figure 3.4D). At this point, the polyp has crossed the line from being benign to being cancerous. Another term for a cancerous tumor that begins in the epithelium (the lining of the intestine and of other tissues such as the throat, urinary tract, or skin) is a *carcinoma*. Malignant tumors that start in the epithelium and contain glandlike tissue are called *adenocarcinomas*.

A carcinoma that remains on the epithelium is sometimes called carcinoma in situ (pronounced "in *sigh*-too"), which, loosely translated, means "a tumor in its original site." Unfortunately, the use of the word "carcinoma" implies that cancer is present. This is somewhat misleading because these polyps are very superficial. They can be easily removed through a simple surgical procedure, resulting in a complete cure. If a doctor tells you that have you carcinoma in situ, don't panic. A few snips of tissue and the problem will go away. Removing adenomatous polyps prevents more than 75 percent of colorectal cancers from developing. After a polypectomy, you will probably be asked to come in for follow-up examinations, during which the doctor will use an endoscope (a viewing device) to make sure that no other lesions are present.

If an adenocarcinoma is left alone, it continues to become more dangerous. It can start to penetrate the deeper layers of the intestine—the muscle layers and eventually the outer layer of the wall (the serosa) (Figure 3.4E and F). Tumors vary widely in size, and more than one tumor can be growing at the same time. Some colorectal tumors grow around the entire circumference of the organ, constricting the intestine like a napkin ring. Others

E   F

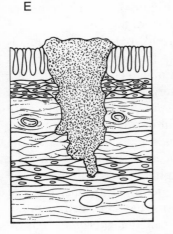
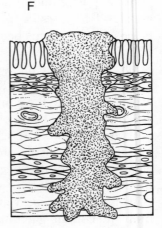

Figure 3.4: Continued.

can push into the open space of the bowel like an expanding bal-
loon. In either path, these tumors can obstruct the bowel and prevent feces from passing through. A tumor may grow so large that
it actually bursts through the organ, spreading cancer into the abdominal cavity.

As they invade the layers of the intestine, cancerous cells can
break free and enter the bloodstream or the lymphatic system,
which carries them to other tissues or organs. Cancer cells in lymphatic vessels travel first to the nearby (regional) lymph nodes and
then to nodes further along the chain (distal nodes). Those that
enter the bloodstream usually travel first to the liver, then to other
sites in the lungs, brain, and bones, where they can cause new tumors to develop. These new tumors are known as secondary or
metastatic adenocarcinomas.

A WORD ABOUT ANAL CANCER

Tumors in the anal region are very different from those in the colon and rectum. Most anal cancers affect only the outer skin. Some tumors may penetrate until they affect deeper layers of skin or other local tissues, but they seldom metastasize to distant locations. They are generally managed the same way as other skin cancers and can usually be treated with drugs, radiation, or surgery.

Anal cancers that involve the cells inside the body, along the anal canal, can penetrate the nearby lymph nodes and are more likely to metastasize. Consequently, they may be more dangerous and harder to treat.

SUMMARY

In this chapter, we looked at what happens inside a cell when cancer strikes and we also defined many important terms. This information may seem technical or confusing at first, but the more you learn about the disease, the better you will recognize how to prevent colorectal cancer and will understand its diagnosis and treatment if it does occur.

Chapter 4

Dietary Strategies for Preventing Colorectal Cancer

By some estimates, about one-third of cancer deaths may be related to improper diet. Strong evidence suggests that, over the long term, making the recommended changes in diet offers a very good chance of reducing the risk of colorectal cancer. A healthy diet may even prove more effective in lowering the death rate from this disease than screening people to find the early signs of cancer or providing treatment for existing cancer.

Given what we know in general about how cancer starts in the body, scientists have good reasons for suspecting that the food we eat plays a role in colorectal cancer. Food particles (or, to be more precise, metabolites—the chemicals in food that are released during digestion) come into direct contact with the mucous membrane that lines the large bowel. As explained in Chapter 3, colorectal cancer begins in the cells that form that membrane. Something causes the cells to change and grow out of control. An irritating substance from digested food is suspected of being that something.

The sequence of eating, digesting, and metabolizing food triggers a series of other events inside the body. (Digestion is the process of breaking food into small parts, or nutrients; metabolism refers to the way the body absorbs, makes use of, or eliminates individual substances.) During digestion of a high-fat meal, for example, the amount of bile released from the gallbladder increases. During metabolism, the presence of certain components of bile (the bile acids) in the chyme may cause cells to grow differently. I'll say a little more about the role of bile later in this chapter.

Food has an impact on the millions of bacteria that live and grow inside the bowel. Bacteria are important in the digestive process because they release enzymes that help break down food. In the process, the bacteria create waste products of their own. The combination of different enzymes and bacterial by-products, in turn, may cause cancerous changes in the cells of the intestines.

Studies of large populations also yield evidence for the impact of diet on colorectal cancer. The food people eat varies greatly from culture to culture, and certain types of diets are clearly associated with lower rates of colorectal cancer. Countries that have adopted the "Westernized" diet show the fastest increases in the rate of this disease. People who move from nonindustrialized countries to industrialized countries, and who adopt the Western diet, are, after just one or two generations, at the same risk of colorectal cancer as the native population.

Still, it is very difficult to identify a specific cause-and-effect relationship between food and colorectal cancer risk. Scientists explore the question from two directions. Their first approach is to look for specific ingredients that might cause cancerous changes in intestinal cells, or that might protect against or neutralize the cancer-causing effects associated with particular foods.

But diets are complex; they involve many foods with dozens of nutrients consumed in different combinations and amounts. For that reason, the second approach is to look at the effects of whole cultural food patterns—what we call diet, or cuisine.

Here's an example of why both approaches are needed in our search for scientific evidence. We know that a diet rich in fiber lowers the risk of colorectal cancer. It would be tempting, therefore, to conclude simply that "fiber prevents cancer." But we get

A FAMILY MATTER

Larry, a 32-year-old printing plant manager, came to see me not ong ago for a diagnostic workup. Larry's mother, age 54, had just learned that she had colon cancer, and Larry was worried that he might be at risk. During the colonoscopic exam, I detected about ten small polyps scattered throughout Larry's colon—enough to indicate that something needed to be done. These polyps had not yet progressed into cancer, but genetic tests showed that Larry was indeed at high risk for the disease. (For more information about this condition, known as hereditary nonpolyposis colorectal cancer, see Chapter 3.) Based on my findings, I explained to Larry my recommendation that he undergo surgery to remove most or, more likely, all of his colon. I also noted that, because his condition was hereditary, there was a good chance his children—two boys, ages 8 and 10—were also at risk. I asked him to make an appointment so that the family could undergo appropriate counseling and some tests.

Larry asked whether his family could do anything to slow down the progression of the disease. I explained to him what we know about the role of diet in reducing the risk of colorectal cancer. Eating foods that are high in fiber and low in fat was the family's smartest move. Basically, this would introduce more fresh fruits and vegetables, more whole-grain foods, and less red meat. I emphasized that these changes were important for Larry's whole family and reminded him that the benefits of a healthy diet included a reduced risk of heart disease and of other life-threatening conditions.

During a follow-up session, I asked Larry how things were going. He said that he and his wife had made a major effort to improve the family diet. "At times, it's been a challenge," Larry said. "The kids were used to having fried chicken or steak for dinner. I admit, we all liked going out for a double cheeseburger now and then. And just try convincing kids that age to eat anything that remotely resembles any shade of green."

Still, he said, they were making progress. "The kids are getting used to the changes we've made," Larry said. "It helped when their mom sat down and explained to them that the doctor said I had a 'tummy problem' and that we all had to be real careful about what we ate. We've discovered lots of ways to make pasta dishes that we can all enjoy. And we've found plenty of good recipes in some cookbooks—most of them aren't too complicated. The other day, it was my turn to do the shopping. Lately, our store has started carrying a lot of ready-made meals that are low-fat or even vegetarian. I was surprised to find that most of these taste pretty good."

fiber by eating vegetables, fruits, and whole grains, which also contain a variety of vitamins, minerals, and other nutrients. The cancer-fighting effect of vegetables may come largely from these substances, individually or in combination, and the fiber may provide other benefits. In addition, there appear to be different effects from the types of fiber that are available. Some studies find that wheat bran fiber protects against colorectal cancer but oat bran fiber does not.

Environmental factors are not the only sources of cancer risk. As mentioned in Chapter 3, some families have a genetic tendency to develop certain forms of colorectal cancer. Within a family, certain individuals inherit genes that may make them more (or less) vulnerable than other family members to the cancer-causing effects of certain foods.

For preventing cancer, the best approach calls for a balanced diet containing a mix of foods eaten in proper proportion. But diet is just one part of an overall healthy lifestyle. Appropriate exercise, moderate (if any) use of alcohol, and no use of tobacco in any form are key components.

In this chapter, I will describe what constitutes a healthy diet and suggest ways to select foods to lower your risk of getting colorectal cancer (and other diseases, for that matter). You will not find it hard or inconvenient to make these important changes in your lifestyle. A wide variety of low-fat, fat-free, or vegetarian foods are available at any grocery store, and many cookbooks offer low-fat recipes that are suitable for the whole family. The next chapter explores the possible benefits of supplementing a balanced diet with substances such as calcium or aspirin. Chapter 11 discusses healthy menus and provides some recipes to help you get started.

If you are interested in lowering your risk of colorectal cancer by making changes in your diet, all of this information should prove helpful.

WHAT IS A DIET?

Today, advertisers bombard us with so much information about diets and nutrition that sorting out the truth from the nonsense can be difficult.

The general term *diet* refers to the usual foods and beverages consumed by an individual or group. When people say they are "going on a diet," they mean that they are making changes in their usual eating patterns, often for medical or health reasons. An acceptable diet must supply three main types of nutrients: (1) fats, (2) proteins, and (3) carbohydrates. Each of these is necessary for the body to carry out its functions.

Fats

Fats are oily nutrients found in a range of foods, including both animal and plant products. The body uses fats to produce the membranes that surround cells, to create certain "working parts" of the cells (known as the organelles), and to produce substances such as steroid hormones. Fats also serve as a source of energy. The body burns fat during times of stress (such as physical activity or emotional tension). Stored fat becomes an emergency energy resource if food supplies run low.

Some of the fatty substances we need are manufactured within the body. Others must be consumed in the diet. Foods high in fat include meats (especially sausage, bacon, and certain cuts of beef); butter, whole milk, and other dairy products; many breads and baked goods; and nuts.

As you probably know, fats are high in calories. A calorie is a measure of energy; specifically, it is the amount of energy needed to raise the temperature of one gram of water by one degree Centigrade. Fat contains nine calories per gram, compared to four calories per gram of carbohydrates or proteins. (One gram is about the weight of a small paper clip.)

Not all fats are created equal. In recent years, such terms as "saturated fat" and "polyunsaturated fat" have become part of our dietary vocabulary. These terms refer to the chemical structure of the fat molecule, which determines how it behaves inside the body. (For the scientifically minded reader: Fats contain atoms of carbon, hydrogen, and oxygen. If the molecule contains high numbers of hydrogen atoms linked to the carbon atom, it is a saturated fat. If there is at least one empty hydrogen "parking space" on the carbon atoms of the fat molecule, it is unsaturated; if there are many such spaces, it is called a polyunsaturated fat.)

Generally speaking, unsaturated fats (such as corn oil) come from vegetables and are liquid at room temperature. Saturated fats (such as butter) come from animal products and are solid at room temperature. Polyunsaturated fats are generally better for health than saturated ones. Monounsaturated fats, such as olive oil, appear to be the best of all. However, foods usually contain several kinds of fat at the same time.

Research shows that fat may contribute to cancer at a number of steps in the digestive process. As mentioned, eating fat causes the body to release bile, which may irritate cells in the colon and trigger abnormal growth. But fat may also play a role in stimulating cells to grow after they have already become cancerous.

Surprisingly, some oils may help protect against cancer. A growing body of evidence suggests that the oils found in fish may help prevent cells in the colon and rectum from becoming cancerous. Researchers have found that a diet of fish oil, which

TRIMMING THE FAT

Here are some suggestions for reducing the amount of fat in your diet.

- Eat meats, especially red meat, less often.
- Choose cuts of meat that are lower in fat. A sirloin steak or beef filet has less fat than a T-bone or prime rib. White poultry meat is lower in fat than dark meat.
- Keep meat servings small. The recommended serving is about three ounces, or a slice about the size of a deck of playing cards—much less than the typical twelve-ounce or sixteen-ounce steak.
- Cut away excess fat before cooking.
- Use skinless chicken.
- Substitute ground turkey for ground beef in meat loaf, tacos, or other such dishes.
- Avoid sausage, bacon, salami, and other processed meats.
- Choose tuna packed in water instead of oil.
- Use nonfat cooking sprays and nonstick cooking utensils to reduce the amount of oil needed during food preparation.
- Select nonfat or low-fat dairy products, including cheese made with low-fat milk.
- Bake, broil, or roast foods instead of frying them.
- Cook meats on racks or grills so that fat can drain away.
- If you travel, request the airline to serve you a low-fat meal.
- Be moderate in your use of mayonnaise, dressings, and similar products that add fat and calories to otherwise healthy salads and side dishes.
- Use nonfat jelly, jam, or fruit spreads instead of butter or margarine.
- Make it a point to read and understand the new "Nutrition Facts" labels now appearing on almost all foods.
   —A product labeled "Fat Free" has less than 0.5 gram of fat per serving.
   —"Low fat" means 3 grams or less.

—Lean means less than 10 grams of fat, including 4.5 grams of saturated fat, and no more than 95 milligrams of cholesterol per serving.

—"Light" (or "lite") means that, compared to the other form of the product, this version has one-third fewer calories, or no more than half the fat, or no more than half the sodium.

—"Cholesterol-free" means the product has no more than 2 milligrams of cholesterol and 2 grams or less of saturated fat per serving.

• Be aware of the fat content of the foods you eat most often, and cut back on the worst offenders.

contains substances called omega-3 fatty acids, seems to block cancer from forming or to slow down the progression of existing colon cancer in laboratory rats. In contrast, diets containing corn oil, safflower oil, or animal fat increased the rate of cancer. More research is needed before we understand the role of fish oil in intestinal disease. Meanwhile, however, it is safe to say that increasing the amount of fish in the diet, especially fish with lower overall fat content, is a good choice, especially as a substitute for red meats or other high-fat foods. Fishes with healthy levels of oil include salmon, swordfish, sole, cod, halibut, trout, flounder, and haddock.

Proteins

Proteins are nutrients that are made up of hundreds, or even thousands, of molecules known as amino acids. (In chemistry, the word *amino* refers to a molecular unit that contains one nitrogen atom and two hydrogen atoms.) The body needs at least twenty different kinds of amino acids to grow and function properly, but it can only manufacture nine kinds. The other eleven, known as essential amino acids, must be consumed in the diet.

During digestion, the protein molecule is broken down into its component amino acids. Our cells can then reassemble the amino acids into various types of new proteins. Fibrous proteins are needed to create skin, hair, nails, muscles, and tendons. Proteins linked with fatty molecules form the membranes that hold individual cells together. Another kind, the globular proteins, can function as hormones, enzymes, and the substances that form the body's immune response against infection. And, some of the amino acid molecules are broken down further and used to build the base molecules that form DNA as the cell reproduces (see Chapter 3). As you can see, proteins are absolutely vital for a healthy, functioning body.

Foods that provide high levels of complete protein (that is, protein that contains all of the essential amino acids) include meat, poultry, fish, eggs, milk, and cheese. Nuts and legumes (peas and beans) contain some but not all of the essential amino acids; these are known as incomplete proteins. Vegetarians—people who do not eat meat—must plan their diets carefully to make sure they eat a combination of vegetables and grains that will supply all the amino acids.

Proteins contain four calories per gram—less than half the calorie content of fat. Excess protein that does not get burned up in the course of a day is stored as fat in the body.

Carbohydrates

Carbohydrates in the diet are the body's main source of energy. Foods that contain sugar, starch, and cellulose are sources of carbohydrates.

There are two kinds of carbohydrates. (1) Simple carbohydrates are basically sugar. They provide calories for energy but not much else in the way of nutrition. Table sugar (sucrose) is an example of a simple carbohydrate. Complex (or unrefined) carbohydrates are supplied by vegetables and cereal grains; they are called complex because they also provide vitamins, minerals, cellulose (fiber), and some protein.

FORMULA FOR A HEALTHY DIET

Despite the confusing information about nutrition, it is possible to plan a diet composed of a good balance of foods, which supplies the needed calories.

Everyone's calorie requirements are different. Highly active people whose jobs entail being on their feet all day will need more calories than sedentary individuals. As a guideline, most Americans probably need around 2,000 calories per day. Table 4.1 shows how these calories should be divided among the major nutrients (fat, protein, and carbohydrates).

On average, no more than 30 percent of a meal's calories should come from fat, and 60 percent should come from carbohydrates. Because fat contains approximately twice as many calories as the other food categories, it takes smaller amounts of fatty foods (by weight) to provide the calories needed. The 30 percent figure is a rough estimate; most people would probably be better off consuming less.

Here's a simple technique for keeping track of how much fat you're getting in a day. Look at the labels on the food packages and find the numbers that represent the percentage of daily value (%DV) for total fat. These percentages, from all the foods you eat in the course of a day, should add up to no more than 100 (100 percent). If you hit that target, you are getting about one-fourth of your daily calorie requirement from fat.

Be aware, however, that the %DV represents the amount of fat *per serving*. A food company's "serving" may not reflect eating habits in the real world. For example, a serving of mayonnaise, defined as one tablespoon, provides 17 percent of the DV of fat. However, a serving of tuna salad made with mayonnaise might easily include twice that amount, or 34 percent of your fat DV—one-third of your daily allotment. You can see how easy it is to eat more fat than you planned.

Another key to healthy eating is not to make yourself crazy over the numbers. What's important is your pattern of eating over the course of time. If you eat above the fat "limit" for one day, eat less the next. The goal is to achieve balance.

TABLE 4.1: RECOMMENDED DIVISION OF CALORIES PER DAY				
Source of Calories	Percentage of Calories	Number of Calories (based on 2000 cal/day)	Calories per Gram	Number of Grams per Day
Fat	20–30%	400–600	9	44–66
Protein	10–15	200–300	4	50–75
Carbohydrates	55–60	1100–1200	4	275–300

Inside the digestive tract, enzymes break complex carbohydrate molecules into simpler forms (called monosaccharides). The main monosaccharides are glucose, galactose, and fructose. In this form, the sugars can be absorbed through the intestines during digestion. They then circulate in the bloodstream to the cells. Some glucose is burned immediately by the cells. The liver converts galactose and fructose into glucose. Glucose that is not burned immediately is converted either to fat or to another substance called glycogen; this excess is stored in the cells for later use. Cellulose, a form of fiber, passes through the body undigested.

Sources of simple carbohydrates include table sugar, syrup, honey, and sweetened foods such as candy and cookies. Sources of complex carbohydrates include whole-grain foods, cereals, fruits, and vegetables such as beans and peas. As noted earlier, carbohydrates supply about four calories per gram.

Other Ingredients

Fats, proteins, and carbohydrates supply us with calories. Foods also contain other essential nutrients; the two main types are vitamins and minerals.

Vitamins are chemicals that serve a number of functions in the body. There are thirteen major vitamins. We need only small amounts of vitamins in our diet, but, like proteins and their amino acids, these are essential for health and well-being. For example, vitamin D is necessary for the formation of bones and teeth. Vitamin D is also significant in a discussion of colorectal cancer because it appears to play a role in protecting the lining of the digestive tract and other tissues in the body. Vitamin E helps keep our cells intact and protects delicate membranes.

Minerals, like vitamins, perform various tasks in the body. At least thirteen minerals are necessary in a complete diet. The most important ones are: potassium, sodium, calcium, magnesium, and phosphorous. Others, such as copper, zinc, and iron, are needed in tiny amounts.

The body cannot manufacture any of the minerals nor most of the vitamins it needs. Instead, we must obtain them through the foods we eat. However, few individual foods can supply all these substances in the proper doses. That's why a balanced diet is so important. Some foods have vitamins or minerals added to them. Milk, for example, contains added vitamin D, and some orange juices contain extra helpings of vitamin C or calcium.

Many people take supplements to make sure they get the full range of vitamins and minerals in adequate doses. In most cases, supplements aren't needed, especially in extremely high quantities, or "megadoses." If you eat proper amounts of a variety of wholesome foods, you'll probably get all the nutrients you need. Also, it is possible to get "too much of a good thing." Overdoses of vitamin A, for example, can cause headache, nausea, diarrhea, liver damage, hair loss, and irregular menstruation. Excessive vitamin C (more than one gram a day) can lead to nausea, stomach cramps, and diarrhea, and too much vitamin D can cause weakness, increased thirst, and gastrointestinal problems.

Recently, other types of nutrients have become the subject of increased interest, especially as possible protections against cancer. One group of these substances, manufactured inside the cells of plants, is called the phytochemicals. Examples of phytochemicals include flavonoids, indoles, and phenols.

Researchers are also investigating a group of nutrients called glucosinolates. Animal studies show that the substance in brussels sprouts that gives them their characteristic bitter flavor can also cause precancerous cells to die before they start growing out of control. A similar substance in broccoli appears to stimulate enzyme activity, which in turn helps neutralize potentially cancerous substances in the colon. Our understanding of these and other plant compounds is in the early stages. It is not possible at this time to identify which of these substances offers the most benefit, and in what amounts. In the future, however, we may see these ingredients listed on food labels alongside a suggested "recommended daily requirement."

Scientists are studying whether the use of food supplements—products such as pills that are not food but contain vitamins and minerals—may play a role in preventing colorectal cancer. That subject is covered in Chapter 5.

FIBER

Fiber, a substance found in plants, helps to hold their cells together. It is not really a nutrient, because it does not get digested (broken down) inside the body. Instead, it passes through the intestine largely unchanged, and that property of fiber makes it a valuable part of a healthy diet.

Fiber appears to protect against cancer in a number of ways. First, it offsets the effects of bile. Bile breaks down into substances called bile acids, such as deoxycholic acid. The presence of these acids can irritate cells and cause them to grow too rapidly, thus raising the risk of cancer. Inside the colon, enzymes acting on the fiber help to neutralize the acidity and offset its impact on cells.

Fiber also helps by absorbing bile acids and carrying them away from the intestinal lining, into the fecal material, and eventually out of the body. One study found that people who consumed two-thirds of a cup of wheat fiber cereal every day for nine months had concentrations of bile acids that were 73 percent lower than those who did not eat fiber.

ANTIOXIDANTS

To carry out their function, the body's cells burn oxygen. During this process, called oxidation, some oxygen atoms undergo a change and become unstable. (To be specific, they lose one of a pair of particles called electrons.) In this state, these unstable atoms, called *free radicals,* are quick to react with other nearby atoms and molecules. Free radicals can damage cells, possibly causing them to become cancerous.

The body doesn't take this kind of insult lying down. It sends other molecules into the area to attach themselves to the free radicals and stop them from doing harm. These chemical white knights are called *antioxidants.* Some of the most important antioxidants are vitamins A, C, and E, and a mineral called selenium. The value of fruits and vegetables as cancer-preventing foods may lie in the fact that they supply the body with chemicals that mop up free radicals.

However, all the facts are not yet in. Despite early enthusiasm for the antioxidant role of beta-carotene (a chemical that the body converts into vitamin A), scientists have not been able to prove those benefits in carefully designed studies in which people took beta-carotene supplements. In fact, beta-carotene appears to *increase* the risk of lung and prostate cancers. Vitamin E (known to scientists as alpha-tocopherol) seems to reduce the risk of prostate and colon cancer, but it may increase the risk of bladder and stomach cancer.

A list of foods that are high in certain antioxidants appears in Table 4.2.

More research is needed before we can state with certainty the relationship among free radicals, cancer, and foods that provide antioxidants.

TABLE 4.2: FOODS RICH IN ANTIOXIDANTS	
Type of Antioxidant	**Foods**
Vitamin A/beta-carotene	broccoli butter cantaloupe carrots egg yolk fortified grain products fortified milk liver margarine peaches spinach squash tomato yams
Vitamin C	broccoli cabbage (raw) cantaloupe citrus fruit and juices (oranges, grapefruit) green peppers kale kiwi spinach strawberries
Vitamin E	dried apricots fortified cereals nuts seeds vegetable and fish-liver oils whole grains

Another way fiber helps is by speeding the passage of feces through the intestine. It appears that the less time digested material stays in contact with the intestinal tissue, the lower the risk of cancer.

Twelve out of thirteen studies conducted recently in nine countries showed that intake of fiber-rich foods significantly lowers the risk of colorectal cancer. Wheat bran and cellulose seem more potent in this regard than oat bran.

How to Get Enough Fiber

The average American consumes perhaps ten grams of fiber a day, but many experts in nutrition advise that the amount should be about three times higher. A good target for daily intake is about thirty-five grams of fiber. If during the course of a day you eat a cup of 100 percent bran cereal, an apple, a potato, and one-half cup of spinach, you will have reached that goal.

If you want to increase fiber consumption, do it gradually, so your body has time to get used to the change. Overdoing fiber consumption (for example, eating up to seventy grams a day) can lead to intestinal cramps, diarrhea, and gas (flatulence). Here are some suggestions:

- Choose whole-grain breads, pastas, and cereals; pass up white flour, white rice, cornmeal, or "enriched" grain products.
- Eat high-fiber cereals, which can provide ten or more grams of fiber in a single serving.
- Snack on fiber bars, air-popped popcorn, or dried fruits (especially apricots and raisins). Nuts have fiber but they are also high in fat.
- Berries—especially those with seeds, such as raspberries or strawberries—are good sources of fiber.
- Eat fruits and vegetables unpeeled, if possible. Apple, cucumber, and potato skins contribute fiber.
- Beans are rich in fiber and can be added to soups, salads, and casseroles.

THE CANCER-PREVENTION SHOPPING BASKET

So far, our diet discussion has focused on what food contains. Let's now look at the foods themselves. We start with vegetables.

The key dietary strategy for preventing cancer of the large bowel is to increase your intake of fresh vegetables and fruits (especially vegetables) while lowering the amount of fat you eat. Vegetables contain many kinds of vitamins and minerals, and hundreds of other nutrients as well. They also supply fiber and very little, if any, fat. If you satisfy your calorie needs through foods derived from plants, you have less need for calories from other, less healthful, sources.

There is mounting scientific evidence that eating vegetables is an effective way to prevent cancer—not just cancer of the colon and rectum, but of the lung and prostate as well. For example, one report on over 750,000 people studied for eight years clearly showed a significant decrease in the risk of colon cancer in men and women whose diets were rich in vegetables. Other studies have reached similar conclusions. Even if colorectal cancer does develop, people who eat cruciferous vegetables—broccoli, cabbage, and the like—seem to have less serious cases of the disease. Other benefits of a vegetable-laden diet include a reduced risk of heart disease, strokes, and diabetes. Recent studies have shown that folate (also called vitamin B12) helps protect against hardening of the arteries.

Vegetables come in many varieties (see Table 4.3). As a rule, green leafy vegetables are the best for you. They supply high quantities of vitamins A and C and moderate amounts of B vitamins, potassium, magnesium, and iron.

Roots and bulbs are good sources of fiber, vitamin C, B vitamins, and minerals, including potassium and magnesium.

The stems and flowers group can supply vitamins A, C, and E, as well as B vitamins, potassium, calcium, and iron.

Beans and peas—often known as legumes—provide a range of important nutrients. Dried varieties (such as pinto and kidney beans) are good sources of iron, calcium, and fiber; fresh legumes have more vitamins, especially vitamins A and C. One important contribution from beans is protein. Beans have been referred to as the "poor man's meat," because they can supply as much protein as beef or chicken. However, as noted earlier, beans don't always provide the full range of amino acids needed for complete

TABLE 4.3: VEGETABLE VARIETIES

Type of Vegetable	Examples
Green leafy	beet greens and turnip greens brussels sprouts cabbage chard collards kale lettuce (especially romaine and endive) spinach Swiss chard
Roots and bulbs	beets carrots garlic onions parsnips potatoes rutabagas turnips
Stems and flowers	artichokes broccoli cauliflower celery leeks
Beans and peas	green beans lentils mung beans navy beans peas pinto beans red beans soy beans
Flowering vegetables	corn eggplant mushrooms peppers pumpkin squash tomato

protein balance. Whole-grain foods, such as wheat and barley, can fill in the gaps. The grains, legumes, and leafy vegetables also supply healthy amounts of folate, which offers protection against colorectal cancer.

Purely in terms of nutrition, the flowering vegetables group is less potent than others, but these foods still offer a fairly good supply of vitamins (especially vitamins A and C) and potassium. Mushrooms (a fungus, a plant that does not contain chlorophyll) are a good source of protein, iron, and B vitamins.

Fruits

Like vegetables, fruits contain a range of vitamins (especially vitamins A and C), minerals (especially potassium), and other nutrients, as well as healthy doses of fiber. Their sweet taste and juicy pulp—plus the fact that they are generally low in calories and sodium—make them a good choice for meals and snacks. Nutritionally speaking, the best fruits are: berries (strawberries, raspberries, and blackberries), persimmons, cantaloupes, mangos, papayas, and dried apricots. The general fruit groups are:

- Seed fruits—apples, grapes, cherries, pears, peaches, apricots, nectarines, and plums.
- Citrus fruits—oranges, lemons, grapefruit.
- Tropical fruits—pineapples, kiwi fruit, papaya, pomegranate.
- Melons—watermelon, honeydew, cantaloupe, casaba.

Grains

Grains are among the oldest and healthiest foods available. The most well-known and widely used grains are wheat, rice, oats, and corn. Other major grains are barley and rye; lesser-known types of flour include buckwheat, soy flour, millet, amaranth, and bulgur.

Grains are used as the basis for flour and are the key ingredients in breads and cereals. However, modern food processing often robs the grain of its healthy properties. Specifically, makers of white flour strip away the outer hull of the wheat kernel, known as the bran, and they remove the inner portion of the kernel, called the germ. They do this so that dough will rise better and will stay fresher on the shelf longer. But bran contributes fiber, and the germ contributes nutrients, including B vitamins, iron, potassium, magnesium, and zinc. Flours, breads, and pastas made with whole grains retain these components and thus generally provide more complete nutrition.

The same is true of rice. All rice starts off brown. In processing, the bran (outer hull) is peeled away, leaving the rice white. Brown rice is much more nutritious than white rice: it contains

TO SERVE AND PROTECT

To guard against cancer, nutritionists recommend eating at least five servings of vegetables and fruits each day. That isn't hard to do, because what counts as a serving is really quite small. Here are some examples of servings:

- $1/2$ cup cooked vegetables
- 1 cup leafy vegetables
- 1 medium potato
- $1/2$ cup of fruit
- $2/3$ cup of fruit juice
- 1 medium apple or orange
- $1/2$ melon or grapefruit
- 1 slice of whole-grain bread
- 1 ounce dry cereal
- $1/2$ cup cooked cereal
- $1/2$ cup rice or pasta

three times the fiber, three to five times as many vitamins, twice as much iron and zinc, and three times the magnesium.

SUMMARY

Colorectal cancer is a highly preventable form of cancer. The key is to eat a combination of foods that provide a variety of nutrients, high levels of fiber, and low levels of fat. By increasing the amount of vegetables and fruits in your diet, and by choosing whole-grain products, you will significantly lower your risk of this disease. In Chapter 11, you'll find some suggested menus, as well as some recipes that will help you achieve these important goals.

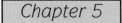

Chapter 5

Other Strategies for Preventing Colorectal Cancer

As you learned in the previous chapter, certain ingredients in the foods we eat offer some degree of protection against cancers of the large intestine. This discovery has led scientists to wonder whether it might be possible to isolate those ingredients and use them, as well as other compounds, to reduce the risk of cancer even further. The strategy of using chemical substances in this way is known as *chemoprevention*. In Chapter 3, I explained how cancer involves changes in cells that occur over long periods of time. Chemoprevention may offer a way to prevent, inhibit, or reverse those changes.

A few cautions. As a science, chemoprevention is still in its infancy. Much more research is needed before we can know precisely what substances will work best, and in what amounts, to lower the risk of colorectal cancer. It is not advisable to rush out and start taking large doses of the substances discussed here.

Also, be careful not to confuse chemoprevention, which is aimed at preventing cancer from developing, with chemotherapy, which is used to treat existing cancer that has invaded nearby or distant tissues.

NSAIDs

A group of medications known as *nonsteroidal anti-inflammatory drugs* (NSAIDs) may play a critical role in preventing colorectal cancer. As their name indicates, NSAIDs relieve inflammation but do so without the use of steroids. NSAIDs are used as pain relievers in the treatment of arthritis, back pain, menstrual pain, headaches, pain after surgery, and soft tissue injuries. Aspirin, the best-known NSAID, also works as a blood thinner; many people take it regularly to reduce the risk that blood clots will form and cause arterial blockage and heart attacks. Other NSAIDs include ibuprofen, sold under the brand names Advil, Motrin, and Nuprin; piroxicam, a prescription medication known as piroxicam (Feldene), used for treatment of arthritis; and sulindac (Clinoril), a prescription NSAID for treatment of arthritis, gout, and other types of joint pain. *

NSAIDs relieve pain by preventing the activity of an enzyme stored inside the cells. Once released, this enzyme, known as prostaglandin H synthetase, attaches itself to a special molecule, known as a receptor, inside the cell. Receptors are like tiny "docking stations." When the enzyme "docks" to the receptor, it triggers changes in the cell's function. One such change involves the release of several chemicals known collectively as *prostaglandins*. These chemicals are responsible for such symptoms as pain and inflammation. They are also involved in transmitting pain signals to the brain.

Prostaglandins are important in a discussion of cancer because they also have various effects on the cell's basic functions. Put simply, some prostaglandins cause cells to grow. They may also cause cells to multiply out of control or to release the energized molecules known as free radicals, which can damage the cell's delicate structure. Prostaglandins also appear to reduce the

---

* Advil: Whitehall-Robins Healthcare; Motrin: McNeil Consumer Products; Nuprin: Bristol-Myers; Feldene: Pfizer; Clinoril: Merck

ability of the immune system to fight off infection. Over time, such changes can contribute to the process by which cells become cancerous. Studies have found, for example, that concentrations of a certain type of prostaglandin (known as PGE2) are higher in adenomatous polyps and adenocarcinomas than in normal tissue. This suggests that these chemical agents may play a role in causing polyps to develop or in converting a benign polyp into a malignant (cancerous) tumor.

NSAIDs may reduce the risk of cancer by causing changes in the cell's enzymes. These changes make it harder for the enzyme to produce potentially harmful prostaglandins that promote cell growth. These drugs may also provide anticancer benefits by enhancing the immune response against cancer cells. Research suggests that NSAIDs may reduce the number of polyps that develop along the intestinal lining. They may also prevent polyps from progressing into cancerous tumors.

Evidence is mounting that NSAIDs do indeed offer protection against cancer. In the 1980s, a study involving over 600,000 adults was conducted by the American Cancer Society. In 1982, the participants reported their frequency and duration of aspirin use. In 1988, the rate and causes of death among the members of this group were studied. Investigators found that the death rate from cancers of the digestive tract, including cancer of the colon and rectum, was about 40 percent lower among people who used aspirin sixteen or more times per month (at least every other day) for a year or more.

Another study involved over 11,000 men and women in Sweden who took NSAIDs for relief of rheumatoid arthritis. Compared to the general population, the NSAIDs group had a 37 percent lower rate of colon cancer and a 28 percent lower rate of rectal cancer. A recent study of people in the health professions noted a 30 percent overall reduction in colorectal cancer, and a 50 percent reduction in advanced cases, among NSAID users. A similar report on 47,000 male health professionals found a lower risk of colorectal cancer among those who used aspirin at least twice a week. A survey of over 47,000 women, conducted by Harvard Medical School, found that those who took four to six aspirin tablets a week for at least ten years had a 44 percent reduction in their risk of colon cancer. Not all such studies have reached the same conclusion, but, overall, the evidence is strong—and growing stronger—that NSAIDs, even in relatively small amounts, provide some benefit.

Other studies are in progress that should help us pin down the right way to use NSAIDs for prevention of colorectal cancer. For example, the Women's Health Study, which involves thousands of female health professionals age forty-five and older, is designed to show whether taking beta-carotene, vitamin E, or aspirin (every other day for four years) has any impact on colorectal cancer.

Like all drugs, NSAIDs cause side effects, some of which are serious. Aspirin can produce ringing in the ears (tinnitus), and it can irritate the lining of the stomach, causing indigestion and nausea. Prolonged use in large doses can lead to bleeding or ulcers in the stomach, as well as problems with blood clotting, liver or kidney damage, and stroke (cerebral hemorrhage). Some people may develop asthmalike reactions. At this time, scientists do not know what doses of aspirin or the other NSAIDs are needed to reduce the risk of colorectal cancer while minimizing the incidence of adverse effects associated with these drugs. A study is under way, for example, that may determine whether 325 milligrams of aspirin each day for four years prevents adenomatous polyps from developing in individuals who have had surgery for early-stage colorectal cancer. Another study is hoping to establish whether very small doses of aspirin (80 milligrams; about one-fourth of the amount contained in a standard tablet) achieve the same results as higher doses.

If you are considering taking aspirin as a preventive strategy, whether for heart attacks or digestive tract cancer, talk to your physician first. At this time, the only aspirin regimen that has received a "seal of approval" from the U.S. Preventive Services Task Force is one aimed at preventing heart attacks. This regimen calls for low doses (one 325-milligram tablet daily or every other day) to be taken by men over age forty who are at significant risk for heart attacks (that is, they are smokers or they have high blood cholesterol, diabetes, or a family history of heart attacks) and who do not have other medical conditions such as bleeding disorders, peptic ulcers, uncontrolled high blood pressure, liver or kidney disease, or stroke. (Results of studies on the use of aspirin for preventing heart problems in women will be available in a few years.) We cannot state with certainty that this same regimen is safe or effective as a method of preventing colorectal cancer.

No drug will work if you do not take it. Sticking with a preventive treatment regimen can be a challenge. In a recent study, participants were paid to take a single aspirin tablet once a day for two weeks. To monitor their compliance, researchers gave them medicine bottles with lids that contained a tiny computer chip that recorded the time of day when they were opened. Even though these participants were paid to take part, only 14 percent of them remembered to take their aspirin tablet at the appropriate time every day throughout the course of the study.

Aspirin works primarily on enzymes of the prostaglandin system. Evidence is mounting that some enzymes of this system are more likely to have a role in promoting colorectal cancer than others. NSAIDs designed to target those enzymes specifically, without affecting the others, may prove to be highly effective in preventing the disease.

For example, ibuprofen, piroxicam, and sulindac block the activity of cyclooxygenase-2, an enzyme involved in the production of prostaglandins. Animal studies suggest that ibuprofen also prevents cells from reproducing abnormally, helps mop up free radicals, and inhibits the development of polyps.

Piroxicam has been found to prevent abnormal cells from developing into cancerous tumors in animals. Studies on humans found that piroxicam in daily doses of 20 milligrams reduced prostaglandin levels by 50 percent in people with a history of adenomas. However, piroxicam can cause side effects such as ulcers or bleeding in the digestive tract. Research is under way to determine whether lower doses of piroxicam, in combination with other cancer-blocking drugs, might be an effective strategy.

Inside the body, the NSAID sulindac breaks down into two different forms, known as metabolites. When given to people with inherited forms of colorectal cancer (such as familial adenomatous polyposis, or FAP), one such metabolite (sulindac sulfide) appears to prevent the development of new polyps or to cause existing polyps to shrink in diameter. The other metabolite, sulindac sulfone, appears to reduce the development of cancerous tumors while posing a lower risk of toxic effects in the digestive system. This substance may also trigger the cell's normal dying process (apoptosis). For these reasons, scientists are very interested in studying whether this form of the drug offers promise as a way to prevent colorectal cancer over the long term.

In addition to its role in inflammation, the prostaglandin PGE2 serves a protective function by stimulating the release of mucus inside the digestive system. Taking NSAIDs reduces this activity, which lowers the mucus level and increases the risk of tissue damage. That's why NSAIDs can cause problems such as bleeding and ulcers. Researchers are hoping to identify drugs that will protect against cancer without robbing the body of the protection offered by PGE2. Similarly, there are two types of the cyclooxygenase enzyme. The goal is to find a medication that will inhibit the cancer-promoting form of the enzyme while leaving the other one alone. Chemicals that achieve this effect have been discovered and are currently being studied. Within the next decade, we should see some exciting developments in this field.

CALCIUM

Another substance that shows some promise as a colorectal cancer preventive is calcium. The body uses this mineral for building bones and teeth. It is also important for the nerves and muscles to carry out their function. The human body contains about two and a half pounds of calcium.

Calcium is needed to maintain the healthy structure of a cell's outer boundary, or membrane. The mineral also plays an important role in transmitting signals to the nucleus, so that cells know when it is time to reproduce, multiply, and die. If disrupted, any of these processes can contribute to the development of cancer.

Looking at data on large populations, scientists noticed that groups of people who consume large amounts of calcium in their diet sometimes show lower rates of colorectal cancer than other groups. Studies in animals show that, during digestion, calcium becomes attached to molecules of fat. This prevents them from being absorbed into the body, thereby reducing the risk that the fat will trigger the abnormal cell growth of cancer. Research also indicates that calcium prevents bile salts, bile acids, and certain enzymes from causing damage to cells—specifically, the cells inside the crypts of the large intestine, where potentially cancerous polyps usually form.

To make use of calcium, the body must maintain adequate supplies of vitamin D. This vitamin helps the intestine to absorb calcium and allows the mineral to pass through the cell walls. Vitamin D comes from such foods as fortified milk, eggs, and seafood. The body also manufactures the vitamin when the skin is exposed to sunlight. Some studies suggest that the cancer-protective value associated with calcium may actually be due to the presence of vitamin D rather than calcium.

As with NSAIDs, we do not yet know what dosage of calcium will offer the greatest amount of protection with the lowest risk of adverse effects. Nutrition experts recommend that adolescents should consume about 1,200 milligrams per day and that older adults need at least 800 milligrams per day. Calcium comes in several forms, some of which may be more readily absorbed than others. Calcium carbonate is the form available in antacid products such as Tums,* which contains 500 milligrams per tablet. Dietary supplements with calcium contain anywhere from 100 to 1,200 milligrams per dose. Before taking calcium products or supplements, talk with your physician, or a nutritionist, about the type and amount that are right for you. Too much calcium can lead to serious health problems, such as kidney stones, and a very recent study suggests that too much calcium (more than 2,000 milligrams daily) may increase a man's risk of developing prostate cancer.

VITAMINS

Chapter 4 discussed the importance of vitamins in a healthy diet. I mention them again here in the context of chemoprevention — the consumption of additional quantities of vitamins specifically as a means of preventing cancer.

Much of the interest in this field has focused on beta-carotene, one of several forms of carotene pigments found in many yellow and dark green fruits and vegetables. Inside the intestine, beta-carotene breaks down into vitamin A (or a form of the vitamin known as retinol). The body needs vitamin A for healthy vision, which is why your mother always told you (correctly) that eating carrots will help you see. The vitamin is crucial for a healthy immune system and is needed for cells to grow normally and maintain their membrane structure and function. Vitamin A also helps absorb and neutralize free radicals, reducing their ability to trigger cancerous changes in cells.

Not long ago, there was a lot of excitement when researchers found evidence that beta-carotene might help protect against certain cancers, such as lung cancer. Unfortunately, subsequent studies found that smokers who took beta-carotene as a single supplement actually developed lung cancer at a higher rate than

* Tums: Smith-Kline Becham

those who took a placebo. It appears that beta-carotene's benefits come only when the substance is consumed as part of a healthy, balanced diet that is low in fat and includes fresh fruits, vegetables, and whole grains.

Evidence that beta-carotene may specifically protect against colorectal cancer is also not very compelling. For example, a recent study of more than 750 patients who had had surgery to remove polyps showed that taking beta-carotene alone or in combination with vitamins C and E for four years did not reduce the rate of growth or the size of adenomatous polyps. Other studies measuring the impact of beta-carotene on different aspects of colorectal cancer development have turned up similarly disappointing results. However, ongoing investigations, such as the Physician's Health Study and the Women's Health Study, are exploring whether different dosages or combinations of treatments will have any impact.

Too much beta-carotene can cause side effects, including headache, nausea, diarrhea, liver damage, hair loss, irregular menstruation, and a yellowish tinge to the skin. Other forms of carotene, such as alpha-carotene, may cause fewer problems and thus may prove to be more beneficial as cancer preventives.

Folic acid, one of the B vitamins, is necessary for making healthy blood cells. People with folic acid deficiency have weaker immune systems, which may increase their risk of various cancers. Studies in both animals and humans have found some evidence that diets high in folic acid (or a related form of the vitamin called folate) may prevent the development of adenomatous polyps in the colon. For example, a study on people with ulcerative colitis, a chronic inflammatory disease that increases the risk of colorectal cancer, found that the incidence of abnormal growths was 2.5 times higher in those who did not take folic acid supplements, compared to those who did. Another study found that people who took sulfasalazine, a drug that interferes with folate absorption and metabolism, had a 50 percent higher risk of growths in the colon compared to those not taking the drug. Scientifically speaking,

these findings are not significant—that is, they might have occurred by chance—and more research is needed to confirm them.
Whether folic acid plays a role in preventing polyps from developing into cancerous tumors has yet to be determined.

Some evidence from studies in rats suggests that vitamin C
may be helpful in keeping polyps from progressing into cancer,
especially in the rectum. Tumors produced experimentally
tended to be less invasive and less likely to metastasize in animals
given vitamin C (ascorbate) than in those fed a normal diet or
given doses of beta-carotene. But again, the difference was not
scientifically significant. In humans, it appears that any benefits
from vitamin C are only part of the picture. Studies on people
treated for adenomatous polyps found that those who took a combination of vitamins A, C, and E for twelve months had a risk of
recurrence of 8 percent, compared to 23 percent for those treated
with lactulose (a sugar derivative) and 41 percent for those who
received no supplements.

Vitamin E is necessary for normal development of the nervous
system, muscles, and blood. It may also lessen the impact of the
natural aging process. Deficiency of vitamin E can cause damage
to muscles, the brain and spinal cord, and can lead to blood disorders such as anemia. As a possible cancer preventive, vitamin E
works to clean up free radicals, maintain the integrity of the cell
membrane, enhance normal cell growth and function, stimulate
the immune system, and prevent excessive cell growth (proliferation). At this time, however, no convincing evidence exists that
taking higher doses of vitamin E than are consumed in a normal
balanced diet will offer any added benefit. Results of some studies
suggest that, just as vitamin D helps the body use calcium, vitamin
E may help by allowing other substances, such as selenium, to
exert anticancer effects.

There are some glimmers of hope that vitamin E may be of
value. A study by the U.S. National Cancer Institute and the National Public Health Institute of Finland found that men who
smoked cigarettes and who were treated for an average of six years
with vitamin E alone or in combination with beta-carotene had

reduced rates of prostate cancer and colorectal cancer (34 percent and 16 percent, respectively). And, as stated above, combinations of vitamins seem to be more effective than vitamin E alone.

HORMONES

A 1995 study, conducted by the American Cancer Society on nearly a half million postmenopausal women, found that use of estrogen in hormonal replacement therapy is associated with a significantly lower risk of death from colorectal cancer. Overall, women who used estrogen replacement therapy at some time in their lives had about half the chance of dying from the disease, compared to those who had never used it. Current users and those who used hormones for a long time (eleven or more years) seemed to benefit the most. It must be pointed out, however, that this study examined only *deaths* from colorectal cancer, not the incidence (number of cases). Scientists are further analyzing the results to determine whether other lifestyle factors, such as healthy diet, exercise, smoking, and level of education, might also be involved. It has been found that use of estrogen for therapeutic purposes is associated with a somewhat increased risk of breast cancer and ovarian cancer. If you are considering extrogen replacement therapy, ask your doctor about the risks and benefits so you can make the choice that's right for you.

OTHER POSSIBLE CHEMOPREVENTIVE AGENTS

Animal studies show that a drug called 2-difluoromethylornithine (DFMO) blocks a crucial step in the proliferation of cells, including cells found in tumors. It also may prevent the process that causes polyps to turn into cancerous tumors. However, DFMO poses a risk of serious side effects, including hearing loss. Research is under way to determine whether this drug is safe for use by humans in a chemoprevention strategy.

Oltipraz is a synthetic substance similar to a compound found in broccoli and other vegetables that is thought to offer some protection against cancer. This drug stimulates the activity of certain enzymes, which may help in the metabolism of fats. Evidence from the laboratory suggests that the drug can block formation of new cancers and that it may also inhibit existing cancers from getting worse. Studies are being conducted to determine whether this is the case in humans.

A number of other chemicals are also under investigation, including a form of bile acid (ursodeoxycholic acid), drugs that inhibit the activity of certain enzymes, and compounds that prevent certain genes from triggering the development of cancerous cells. However, it will be years before we have conclusive proof that any of these are of value as methods of preventing colorectal cancer.

SUMMARY

At this time, it is not possible to state conclusively that taking special dietary supplements, vitamins, or drugs will offer any real protection against the growth of colorectal polyps or their progression into cancerous tumors. The National Cancer Institute and the American Cancer Society both recommend that people avoid taking large doses of vitamins, minerals, or other such agents unless they are taking part in a study or are under the careful supervision of a physician. Undoubtedly, in the next few years, we will see some exciting developments in this field—developments that promise to reduce the incidence of the disease and the suffering it can cause.

What can be said without qualification, however, is that the best way to reduce the risk of colorectal cancer—and a host of other diseases, for that matter—is to use common sense: eat a healthy, balanced, low-fat diet with lots of fresh vegetables and fruits; avoid tobacco; reduce alcohol intake; and exercise regularly.

Chapter 6

Screening and Early Detection

The use of diet, supplemental vitamins, or other substances to prevent cancer from developing is known as *primary prevention*. The focus of this chapter is *secondary prevention* — the methods doctors use to discover polyps before they become cancerous, or to identify cancer in the early stages, before it grows and spreads. Research shows that the suffering caused by colorectal cancer could be significantly reduced by wider use of secondary prevention.

The two main strategies for secondary prevention are screening and early detection. *Screening* means taking steps to look for a disease even when there's no obvious reason to suspect that a person might have it. Screening can also be done in people who are at higher-than-average risk of colorectal cancer, such as those with a family history of the disease. *Early detection* means diagnosing the disease at an early enough stage so that treatment can produce the best possible outcome, including a complete cure.

The main tests that are used to achieve secondary prevention are:

- Digital rectal examination (DRE).
- Fecal occult blood test (FOBT).
- Flexible sigmoidoscopy (use of a viewing scope to see inside the lower part of the large bowel).
- Colonoscopy (use of a scope to view the entire large bowel).
- Double contrast barium enema (an X-ray test to view the lining of the large intestine).

These strategies can be effective because of the nature of colorectal cancer. As you learned in Chapter 3, it takes years—often a decade or more—for a polyp to grow and progress into a cancer. Identifying and removing those abnormal tissues (also called lesions) before they can become cancerous, or identifying cancer before it spreads to other parts of the body, is essential.

Many intestinal lesions do not cause any symptoms, especially in the early stages. The ability to detect cancer at this point is the biggest single factor in calculating the odds for long-term survival. Up to 90 percent of people whose colorectal cancers are discovered and treated in the early stages will live for ten years or more. In contrast, only about 5 percent of people whose colorectal cancer has spread to the liver will survive five years or more.

Screening is a controversial subject in medicine because it means subjecting people to tests even when there is no apparent reason for suspicion. It adds to the nation's total health care bill and causes patients some degree of inconvenience and discomfort. Certain screening procedures, such as sigmoidoscopy, are invasive, and they carry some risk in themselves. However, screening for a disease is justified when:

1. The disease is common.
2. The illness is associated with serious risk of disability and death.
3. The screening tests available are sufficiently accurate to detect a disease early enough to justify treatment.
4. The tests are acceptable to patients.
5. The tests can be conducted safely in a general medical practice.
6. Treatment improves the outcome (prognosis).
7. Potential benefits outweigh the risks and costs.

Screening for colorectal cancer meets these guidelines. This form of cancer is certainly common—it is the second leading cause of cancer deaths in both men and women. Early detection

provides an opportunity to treat the disease effectively, often producing a cure and adding years, even decades, to a person's life.
Careful research has shown that a combination of screening tests,
if properly chosen and administered, allows accurate detection of
early-stage colorectal cancer. These tests also identify noncancerous polyps that can be removed, thereby reducing the risk that
they will develop into cancer. The benefits of these procedures
far outweigh any risks they might pose.

Today, the rate at which people actually get screened is on the
increase, but the overall numbers are still relatively low. A nationwide study in 1993 found that 43 percent of respondents had had
a DRE during the preceding year, and 28 percent had had a sigmoidoscopy at some point during the preceding five years. Men
were more likely than women to have had a sigmoidoscopy (33
percent and 24 percent, respectively) and to have had a DRE (47
percent and 40 percent, respectively). Whites were more likely
than African Americans to have had a sigmoidoscopy (29 percent
and 26 percent, respectively) and to have had a DRE (44 percent
and 39 percent, respectively). Age is also a factor: 23 percent of
persons aged fifty to fifty-nine years had a DRE, and 32 percent
of persons aged seventy years or older had received this test.

Personal income and level of education are factors that affect
the extent of screening. Among people who responded to the 1993
survey and who earned less than $15,000 annually, 35 percent re-
ported a DRE, and 24 percent reported a sigmoidoscopy; among
those earning more than $50,000 a year, 55 percent reported a
DRE, and 35 percent reported a sigmoidoscopy. Among those
with less than twelve years of education, the rates for DRE and sigmoidoscopy were 37 percent and 24 percent, respectively. The
rates rose among those with a college education: 49 percent reported a DRE, and 32 percent reported a sigmoidoscopy.

An increase in the extent of screening will require raising public
awareness of its benefits. This book is part of that effort. Also, in
1997, a nationwide group of interdisciplinary physicians and other
health care experts concerned about colorectal cancer published a

report on the importance of being tested for the disease. Their findings, which are reflected in the discussion that follows, were endorsed by a number of professional associations, including:

- American Cancer Society.
- American College of Gastroenterology.
- American Gastroenterological Association.
- American Society of Colon and Rectal Surgeons.
- American Society for Gastrointestinal Endoscopy.
- The Crohn's and Colitis Foundation of America.
- The Oncology Nursing Society.
- Society of American Gastrointestinal Endoscopic Surgeons.

In this chapter, I'll describe some of the tests and procedures used to screen for colorectal cancer. Other procedures, including colonoscopy and the double contrast barium enema, are discussed in the following chapter, which deals with the diagnosis of cancer.

Keep in mind that each of the secondary prevention methods described here has advantages and disadvantages. To get the most

---

AMERICAN CANCER SOCIETY COLORECTAL CANCER SCREENING GUIDELINES

Beginning at age fifty, both men and women should follow this testing schedule:

- Yearly fecal occult blood test (FOBT), plus flexible sigmoidoscopy every five years, or
- Colonoscopy every ten years, or
- Double contrast barium enema every five to 10 years.

A digital rectal exam should be done at the time of each sigmoidoscopy, colonoscopy, or barium enema.

AMERICAN CANCER SOCIETY SCREENING GUIDELINES FOR PEOPLE AT HIGH RISK

Risk Factor
Family history of familial adenomatous polyposis (FAP)

Screening Recommendations
Genetic counseling.
Consider genetic testing.
Flexible sigmoidoscopy annually, beginning at puberty.
Consider colectomy if polyps are detected.

Risk Factor
Family history of hereditary nonpolyposis colorectal cancer (HNPCC)

Screening Recommendations
Genetic counseling.
Consider genetic testing.
Colonoscopy every one to two years starting between ages twenty and thirty, and every year after age forty.

Risk Factor
Relative (parent, sibling, child) who has colorectal cancer or adenomatous polyps

Screening Recommendations
Same as for average-risk individuals, but beginning at age forty.
Especially important if the relative had colorectal cancer before age fifty-five or adenomatous polyps before age sixty.

Risk Factor
Personal history of inflammatory bowel disease, including ulcerative colitis or Crohn's disease

Screening Recommendations
Complete colonoscopy every one to two years after eight years of disease (after fifteen years if only the left colon is involved).

Risk Factor
Previous colon cancer

Screening Recommendations
Colonoscopy one year after surgery; if normal, repeat after three years.
If repeat colonoscopy is normal, repeat every five years thereafter.

Risk Factor
History of adenomatous polyps

Screening Recommendations
Colonoscopy one year after polyps first detected.
Repeat colonoscopy in three to five years if first follow-up is normal or if only a single small adenoma is found.
Repeat more often if numerous adenomas, large sessile adenomas, or polyps with invasive cancers are found.

complete and accurate picture, you need to combine several of the methods. Also, in most cases, a positive result on one or more screening tests is an indication that further tests are needed to diagnose or rule out the presence of cancer.

Which of these tests are given, when, and how often depends on whether you are at average risk or high risk. Average risk basically includes all men and women over the age of fifty. About 75 percent of all new cases of colorectal cancer occur in people who have no known risk factors other than age. People at high risk for colorectal cancer should be screened earlier and more often, using the full range of available tests and procedures, including colonoscopy. However, if only people who are at high risk are screened, doctors will miss detecting a large majority of cancers in the large intestine.

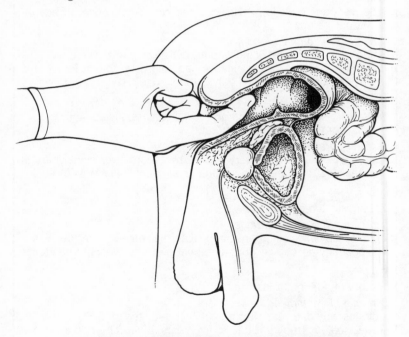

Figure 6.1: Digital rectal examination (DRE).

DIGITAL RECTAL EXAMINATION (DRE)

The DRE is a common procedure performed during a routine medical examination (Figure 6.1). The physician puts on a glove, applies a lubricant, inserts a finger into the rectum, and feels around for any unusual growths. The procedure is not usually painful, although it may be somewhat uncomfortable. The DRE can reveal the presence of polyps or other growths in the anus and rectum.

The DRE is an important part of an annual checkup for everyone, especially people over the age of fifty. In men, the DRE can often detect cancerous lumps or nodules in the prostate, a male sex gland. In women, the procedure can identify unusual growths or other problems in parts of the pelvic region.

Although it is useful in screening for colorectal cancer, the DRE is not complete by itself. Part of the reason is anatomical. The large intestine is about five feet long, and a finger is only about four inches in length. Only about one in four intestinal cancers or adenomatous polyps will develop in the rectum. So, at best, the DRE cannot detect problems in the majority of the organ. Also, this is a "blind" procedure. The physician cannot see what is being felt. An unusual lump or growth may be a polyp or a cancer, or it may be some other abnormal but nonthreatening tissue. The DRE does not always identify all the lesions that may be present. To some extent, too, the effectiveness of the test depends on the thoroughness and experience of the examiner.

Overall, the DRE by itself might detect approximately 5 to 10 percent of colorectal cancers or adenomatous polyps—enough to make this a useful but insufficient first step.

FECAL OCCULT BLOOD TEST (FOBT)

Polyps and cancerous tumors often cause bleeding in the intestine. About two-thirds of cancers bleed in the course of a week.

Polyps are less likely to bleed, but the larger the lesion, the greater the chance that bleeding will occur.

Some of this blood is carried out of the body in the feces. Because the amount of blood may be relatively small, it may not be visible to the eye. It is hidden—or, in scientific language, "occult."

The fecal occult blood test (FOBT) is a simple, convenient, and inexpensive method for identifying this hidden blood. The most commonly used brand of FOBT is Hemoccult II. A small smear of feces is placed in several spots on a piece of test paper that has been soaked with a chemical and mounted in a cardboard frame. The examiner then applies another chemical (hydrogen peroxide) to the paper. This fluid reacts with the fecal material. If blue spots show up, it means blood is present in the feces.

Many physicians perform an FOBT immediately after the DRE, since fecal material is present when the gloved finger is removed. However, because not all intestinal lesions bleed all the time, a single test may not detect bleeding on a particular day. In fact, the test is not designed to be used in that manner. The best results come from doing the test at home, collecting three separate stool samples over the course of three days. Cards containing the sample are sealed and delivered to the analyzing lab, either in person or by mail.

American Cancer Society guidelines call for doing FOBT every year for people who choose flexible sigmoidoscopy plus FOBT from among the three colorectal cancer screening options. Annual FOBT may detect lesions that were missed on earlier rounds of screening but are still in an early enough stage that treatment can provide a cure. Overall, the FOBT produces positive results (that is, it detects bleeding) in about 2 to 6 percent of patients. Subsequent tests on people who have positive FOBT results will detect cancerous growths (carcinomas) in about 5 to 10 percent, and adenomas (noncancerous growths that may develop into cancer) in 20 to 40 percent.

Studies show that, when used properly in colorectal cancer screening programs, annual FOBT tests offer a greater than 70 percent chance that an existing tumor will eventually be detected. When a positive test for fecal occult blood is followed by complete diagnostic evaluation of the colon—and treatment, if cancer is found—the risk of death from colorectal cancer is significantly reduced. This approach detects cancers at earlier stages and increases the length of survival time.

No test works, however, unless it is performed. A study in the mid-1980s found that only about half of physicians follow the ACS recommendations for using the FOBT. And patients are often remiss in completing the test at home, collecting stool samples over the course of one to three days. For example, one study found that up to 80 percent of examinees complied with the FOBT process the first year, but only about 16 percent were still complying after two years. People who are aware of the risks of colorectal cancer—those who have friends or family members with the disease, for example—are more likely to comply. Some people resist doing the test because they are not being bothered by any symptoms, even though colorectal cancer is often symptomless. Others resist because of the embarrassing or unpleasant nature of the test or because they do not want to know that they might have a health problem. With colorectal cancer, however, what you don't know can definitely hurt you.

With growing public awareness of the importance of this disease, and since the recent publication of the interdisciplinary panel's report on the need for screening, use of FOBT will no doubt become more widespread.

I strongly advise against using the home FOBT tests that now available for purchase at a pharmacy. Because of many problems with such tests, they are not recommended.

Limits of the Test

There are some limits to the usefulness of the FOBT. For example, everybody loses a little blood in the intestine—an average of about 2 milliliters (mL) per day. For the FOBT to be accurate (that is, to detect blood loss from a disease rather than from the normal process of digestion), the rate of blood loss must be at least 20 mL per day. But polyps or cancer can exist without producing that degree of bleeding. Thus, the FOBT may result in an "all-clear" result when bleeding (and possibly cancer) is actually present. Such results are known as *false negatives*. The false negative rate with the FOBT is as high as 50 percent for carcinomas and 70 percent for adenomas.

FOBT is not an invasive test, and there are no complications or risks involved. One concern, however, is that false positive results (that is, a test showing that bleeding is occurring when in fact it is not) generate unnecessary anxiety, and false negative results produce unwarranted reassurance that everything is fine.

The size of the lesion is also a factor. Polyps or cancerous lesions less than 1 or 2 centimeters (cm) in diameter are less likely to bleed. Also, lesions in the left (descending) colon are more likely to produce positive tests than those in the right (ascending) colon.

FOBT is not a specific test for colorectal cancer; it may detect blood from causes other than polyps or cancer, such as gum disease, gastritis, peptic ulcer disease, or hemorrhoids.

As noted earlier, the timing of the test and the amount of bleeding also affect results. A tumor may bleed at some times and not at others, or the rate of bleeding may fluctuate over time. If the FOBT happens to be done at a time of low flow, the results may not reflect the true state of affairs. For this reason, doctors often urge patients to conduct the FOBT at home over the course of three days. A single positive result from any of the samples indicates the need for further tests.

It is also important to have the results analyzed promptly, because tests analyzed after more than four days are more likely to generate false negatives. Additional tests usually need to be done at home, and the test cards should be sent to the processing lab without delay.

The foods consumed just prior to the test can also make a difference. Vitamin C (ascorbic acid) can mask the presence of bleeding and produce a false negative test. On the other hand, salicylate drugs (such as aspirin) and foods such as turnips, horseradish, broccoli, cauliflower, radishes, rare red meat, cabbage, potatoes, cucumbers, mushrooms, and artichokes can cause false positive reactions (in other words, the results indicate bleeding when no bleeding is occurring). Taking iron tablets can turn the stool dark, making it difficult to interpret the blue color change of a positive test. If you are scheduled for an FOBT, avoid the foods mentioned and do not take iron supplements a few days before, or during, the days of the test.

Remember that FOBT is only a screening test that offers an indication of the possible presence of cancers and large polyps. The test is not a substitute for a precise diagnosis. Any positive results on FOBT are a sign that the person should undergo further diagnostic studies, including double contrast barium enema with or without flexible sigmoidoscopy, or colonoscopy. In this regard, false positives can be a blessing in disguise. Even though such results wrongly indicate that bleeding is occurring, they often lead to further testing that reveals the presence of polyps or cancers, even though these lesions were not actually bleeding at the time of the original test.

FLEXIBLE SIGMOIDOSCOPY

In the past few decades, advances in medical technology have led to the development of smaller and more accurate viewing instruments that physicians can use to peer deeper inside the body than ever before. Instead of having to rely on indirect or incomplete observations, or the results of laboratory tests, today it is possible to get a direct look at the site of the problem. This in turn leads to more precise diagnosis and more specific and effective treatment.

In the realm of colorectal cancer, one major leap forward has been the development of the flexible sigmoidoscope, a viewing instrument that is inserted into the anus. A light source attached to the scope illuminates the area and gives the physician a good look at the tissue. Because it is flexible, it can be manipulated around the twists in the large intestine, specifically in the sigmoid (S-shaped) part of the lower colon. Today, the instrument used most often has a viewing range of up to 60 centimeters (cm; about 27 inches). Another model has a range of 35 cm. The 60-cm flexible sigmoidoscope (or "flex sig") is a great improvement over the previous model, the 20-cm rigid sigmoidoscope, first developed in the mid-1950s. Because the rigid scope was only one-third the length of the flexible version, it did not permit as great a range of vision. And because it was rigid, it was more likely to cause pain. Today, most endoscopists (physicians who specialize in this procedure) use only the longer flexible version.

The flexible sigmoidoscopy can be done in a physician's office without the need for anesthesia. The procedure itself takes about eight to ten minutes (up to twenty minutes in some cases). However, it is necessary to prepare for the procedure by undergoing one—or, in most cases, two—enemas to cleanse the bowel. The Fleet enema, a liquid solution that comes in a squeezable plastic container, is one of the most commonly used brands. You insert the nozzle of the container into the rectum and squeeze the liquid into the bowel. The liquid contains a chemical that stimulates a bowel movement. You should hold the liquid in as long as possible, until the urge to have a movement becomes irresistible. In the doctor's office, you may be asked to undergo a second enema. If you are unable to do the enemas yourself, the office staff will offer to help you.

The flexible sigmoidoscopy is a very safe procedure. However, you may be given an antibiotic if you are at risk of heart infections (endocarditis) or if you have had heart valve or other open-heart operations.

As you lie on your side, the physician inserts the scope through the anus and maneuvers it as far into the colon as possible, examining the tissue along the way. The procedure is not painful but may it produce some discomfort. Most people describe the discomfort as mild, but for about 10 to 15 percent of patients, it is moderate. Afterward, the physician will discuss the results with you and will advise you whether any additional tests or procedures are necessary. The presence of any cancer or of a polyp larger than 1 cm is usually considered a positive result. Some physicians also consider that the presence of any adenoma, regardless of size, requires a more extensive workup.

If the examiner detects a polyp, the lesion can be biopsied during the sigmoidoscopy. A biopsy involves removing a portion of the growth and sending it to a laboratory for analysis. Biopsies that turn out to contain only normal tissue or hyperplastic (noncancerous) growth do not require follow-up. However, if the polyp turns out to be adenomatous (precancerous) or cancerous, then the physician will usually recommend that you have a colonoscopy so that the entire colon can be studied. Polypectomy—complete removal of polyps—is not performed during the sigmoidoscopy. Such a procedure is handled separately, after a complete bowel cleansing. The device for conducting a polypectomy, called an electrocoagulator, uses heat and electricity to remove the lesion. The instrument then seals off the tissue to promote healing.

Sigmoidoscopy is a very valuable tool in the colorectal cancer screening and prevention process. A study on 26,000 people who underwent the procedure (using a rigid scope) at a clinic in New York turned up 58 cases of colorectal cancer—one for every 450 people screened. Eight out of 10 of those detected were in the early stages (Stage I or II), when treatment offers the best hope for cure. About 80 percent of those patients were still alive fifteen years after detection and treatment. Another study (also involving the rigid sigmoidoscope) looked at 5,000 patients, only some of whom had the sigmoidoscope exam. In the sixteen years of the study, there were twelve deaths from colorectal cancer among those who had had the sigmoidoscope exam and twenty-nine deaths among those who did not—a risk reduction of nearly 60 percent. A third investigation (involving both rigid and flexible scopes) reported that the risk of fatal colon cancer was decreased by 60 to 80 percent among individuals who had undergone one or more sigmoidoscopic examinations, compared to a group of patients who did not receive screening.

Using a computer-generated statistical model, scientists have predicted that, in a population of 100,000, performing sigmoidoscopy every five years would reduce the incidence of colorectal cancer from about 5,000 to about 3,000 cases, or 40 percent. The number of deaths from colorectal cancer would also decrease proportionately. The average life expectancy of people whose deaths from the disease were prevented by using this approach would be increased by nearly nine years.

The implication is clear: Use of the scope increases the chance that cancer will be detected at an early stage, thus improving the opportunity for treatment, cure, and long-term survival. Current screening guidelines urge that people over the age of fifty should undergo a sigmoidoscopic exam every five years. This time interval reflects the nature of the disease: polyps are not likely to arise and progress to advanced cancer within a five-year period.

Some risk is associated with any invasive procedure, and the sigmoidoscopy is no exception. Infection can develop. There is a slight chance—about 1 to 3 in 10,000—that the scope may perforate the bowel wall. Often, this problem can be corrected with a few stitches and is not always serious, but the patient must be sent to a hospital (the sigmoidoscopy is usually done in a doctor's office). Serious bleeding can develop in about 10 out of 10,000 cases. There is also a slight risk of death.

Using the flexible sigmoidoscope, a physician can see the whole sigmoid colon in about 80 percent of cases. Because approximately 50 to 60 percent of cancers and adenomas occur in this region, the procedure has a chance of detecting between 40 and 60 percent of any lesions present. (In contrast, the rigid instrument could discover only about 25 to 35 percent of polyps.) Still, a significant number of all colorectal cancers and polyps will not be spotted. This is a concern because the presence of one polyp in the rectum or sigmoid colon may indicate that another one is present elsewhere in the bowel, possibly beyond the reach of the sigmoidoscope. For that reason, a positive finding during this procedure usually means that a colonoscopy is also needed, not just to remove the known lesions but to look for others farther up inside the intestine. By the same token, about one in three patients in whom sigmoidoscopy finds no lesions do in fact have lesions in the farther reaches of the bowel.

The combination of annual fecal occult blood tests plus sigmoidoscopy every five years offers an excellent chance of detecting colorectal cancer in the early stages. Evidence to support this conclusion can be found in a study showing that two-thirds of the cancers missed by FOBT were detected through the use of flexible sigmoidoscopy. Another study found that the death rate from colorectal cancer in patients screened with FOBT plus sigmoidoscopy was 36 per 1,000, compared to 63 per 1,000 in a group screened with sigmoidoscopy only.

COLONOSCOPY AND DOUBLE CONTRAST BARIUM ENEMA

Until recently, the American Cancer Society's recommendation for colorectal cancer screening was yearly digital rectal examination and FOBT, and flexible sigmoidoscopy every five years. In 1997, the ACS revised these recommendations. The combination of digital rectal exam, FOBT, and sigmoidoscopy is still approved as one of the three options for screening. The second option is colonoscopy and digital rectal exam every ten years. The third option is double contrast barium enema and digital rectal exam every five to ten years. The FOBT is used in combination with the sigmoidoscopy because the sigmoidoscopy does not permit examination of the entire colon. Because colonoscopy and double contrast barium enemas examine the entire colon, FOBT is not needed. Besides being on the list of screening tests, colonoscopy and double contrast barium enema examinations

FIRSTHAND EXPERIENCE

"I admit, I was pretty upset about the thought of undergoing a sigmoidoscopy," said Jeanette, a 60-year-old elementary school principal. "I really didn't relish the thought of lying on an operating table with my backside exposed while a bunch of strangers poked a tube into me. And I was pretty surprised when the doctor told me I wouldn't need anesthesia for the procedure. He said it wouldn't be painful. Maybe not, but I was secretly hoping they would just knock me out and I could wake up when this humiliating business was all over.

"As it turned out, it wasn't as quite as bad as I had thought. No day at the beach, but not exactly the nightmare I'd feared.

"The first thing I had to do was give myself an enema. The nurse at the doctor's office had offered to handle the enema for me if I didn't want to. But I preferred to do it at home, and I figured out how to do it without much hassle. You kneel on the floor and inject the contents of a flexible bottle into your bottom. A few minutes later I had a powerful bowel movement. I then drove myself to the doctor's office, where they asked me to do a second enema. By then I felt like an experienced pro.

"Then it was time for the sigmoid exam itself. The doctor showed me the scope and explained how it worked. It looked like a short black garden hose, only not as big around, and it had a little lens on the tip. Then the nurse asked me to lie on my left side, lifted my examining-room gown, and applied some kind of lubricant. I had to remind myself that these are professionals, they're used to this sort of thing. The doctor then began inserting the scope. I gritted my teeth and tried to grin and bear it—without the grinning. It felt very strange—the opposite of having a bowel movement. Instead of feeling stuff passing *out* of my body, I felt something passing *in*. It was uncomfortable, and the thought of it all was pretty repugnant. But to my surprise it was not really painful at all.

"I did what I could to distract myself. I was facing a blank wall, and there wasn't much to look at. So I closed my eyes and tried to think about pleasant scenes—my trip to Tuscany two years ago; my last visit with my granddaughter; the surprise party my husband staged for me on my sixtieth birthday. I softly hummed a little tune to help drown out the sounds of the examining room. I counted the number of times I breathed. For the record, it was 230. It's strange, but during procedures like this you can talk yourself into having a kind of 'out-of-body' experience—imagining that you're a thousand miles away.

"Fortunately, the procedure was over in less than eight minutes. I felt the tube being withdrawn—for one embarrassing moment, I thought I was having an accidental bowel movement, until I remembered that after those two enemas there wasn't much left inside me to move.

"Afterward, I met with the doctor, who explained what he had found—or rather, what he hadn't found. There were no signs of polyps or other problems. That feeling of reassurance was a pretty good tradeoff for having to put up with the procedure. In five years, when I have to subject myself to this process again, I'll know what to expect. I'll be able to get through it with a lot less anxiety and dread."

are often used as diagnostic tests. They are discussed in detail in Chapter 7.

OTHER TESTS FOR EARLY DETECTION

Blood Tests

Recently, some new variations on the fecal occult blood test have appeared on the market. One of these, Hemoccult II Sensa, is designed to be more sensitive than its predecessor. Another test, HemeSelect, reacts with a different component found in the blood (hemoglobin). These or future tests may prove to be more precise in identifying bleeding caused by cancers in the lower digestive tract. Unlike Hemoccult, these tests do not require dietary restrictions or avoidance of medications before they can be given. They are also more expensive.

At this time, studies have not been done to confirm that the new tests offer advantages over existing methods, but there is reason to be optimistic.

Tumor Markers

Cancerous cells produce certain substances, including enzymes and proteins called antibodies, and release them into the bloodstream. Like footprints left behind by a thief, these substances, known as tumor markers, provide telltale clues of the presence of cancer and the nature of a tumor. Laboratory tests can sometimes be developed to identify these substances. Also, sensitive molecular tests can detect the presence of abnormal genes in the feces.

Scientists are also trying to develop a blood test that identifies colon mucoprotein antigen, a form of protein that is produced only by colon cancer tumors.

Virtual Colonoscopy

Recently, a new medical device has been developed that works like the computed tomography (CT) scan to create three-dimensional images of the entire intestine. As the patient lies on a table, the machine spins around the person's body in a spiral pattern. Precisely focused rays are emitted that bounce off the tissues. The computer calculates the data and generates the picture. The observer can then view the image on a monitor and navigate through it as though using a colonoscope.

The procedure, known as a virtual colonoscopy, is still in its fledgling stages. The technology is expensive and is not yet widely available. But it may become a useful alternative to other screening methods. One potential advantage is its quickness — the patient is inside the machine for only a minute or so. As is the case with a true colonoscopy, bowel cleansing is needed to remove material from the intestine, but the procedure itself is not invasive—no fingers or scopes are inserted into the anus. Also, it allows a view of the entire intestine, not just the rectum and sigmoidal colon, as is the case with the sigmoidoscope. Research is needed to determine the procedure's accuracy for detecting small lesions or identifying dangerous cancers. But there is hope that such a method will increase the ability to detect and treat colorectal cancer at an earlier stage than ever before.

Chapter 7

Diagnosis

As explained in the previous chapter, screening for colorectal cancer occurs when doctors look for the disease in people who have no symptoms. Colorectal cancer screening includes people without any known risk factors as well as those who may be at high risk because of a hereditary tendency to develop colon polyps.

Diagnosis is a different process. In making a diagnosis, physicians conduct more extensive tests to:

1. Establish that a disease is definitely present,
2. Give it an accurate name,
3. Distinguish it from other similar conditions, and
4. Plan the types of treatment needed.

Understandably, receiving a diagnosis of cancer is a terribly upsetting experience, not just for the person with the disease but for the family and friends as well. Often, when people hear they have cancer, they imagine they are doomed to suffer pain and debility for the rest of their lives. Many believe they have been handed a death sentence.

I'd like to offer you reassurance. In one important way, receiving a diagnosis, even of a frightening disease such as cancer, can be seen as a positive step. Your doctors have identified the problem and can begin taking the action needed to help you. Modern treatment for colorectal cancer offers strong hope for a complete recovery that can add years of fully functional life. I'm not saying that coping with the illness and its treatment is without risks or difficulties. My point, instead, is to emphasize that healing can only begin when the problem has been identified—when a diagnosis has been made.

When detected early and treated promptly, cancer of the colon and rectum is one of the most curable forms of the disease. Over three-fourths of people with this form of cancer can be cured. Nearly 75 percent of those with local cancer (Stage I or II) will survive at least ten years after their diagnosis, and nearly 50 percent of those with Stage III will survive five years or more. Because colorectal cancer develops over a long period of time, it is possible to detect the disease long before symptoms appear. Early detection of small cancers also reduces the likelihood of having to undergo major surgery.

WHAT SYMPTOMS TELL US

Often, the diagnosis of colorectal cancer occurs because the person notices troubling symptoms. However, the optimal time for a diagnosis of this disease is in the earliest stages, before any symptoms develop. Because colorectal cancer arises inside body organs that are hidden from direct observation, a tumor can progress for a long time, even years, before it might be noticed. When symptoms do arise, it is often because the cancer has become so large that it is blocking the intestine or because it has already spread to other tissues or sites in the body. Treatment is still possible at this stage, but it is more complex and less certain to result in a cure. The earlier the cancer is detected, the more hopeful the prognosis or outlook for the future. That's why it's so important to see a doctor if you notice rectal bleeding or any other potential signs of the disease.

Chapter 3 described the common symptoms of colorectal cancer: a change in bowel habits—more frequent or less frequent

bowel movements, a change in the shape or consistency of stool—
and other problems such as bleeding and abdominal pain. The
exact types of symptoms that develop give some clues about the location and the extent of the tumor. As you read the following para-
graphs, you might want to look again at Figure 2.1, on page 18, to
remind yourself of the anatomy.

When digested food (chyme) leaves the small intestine, it passes
through a valve and enters the first part of the large intestine (the
cecum, located in the right, or ascending, colon). If the valve is
damaged (whether by cancer or by some other problem, such as
Crohn's disease), the chyme may become blocked, resulting in obstruction in the small bowel. Patients with this condition will experience cramps and swelling of the abdomen. Some may also
experience nausea. They may vomit a substance that is grayish-
green in color because it contains large amounts of the digestive
fluid called bile.

As chyme flows into and up the right side of the large intestine,
it is still in a very liquid state. The colon is quite wide at this location. Because chyme can still flow through the organ, any
tumor that develops here will cause intestinal blockage only if it
grows very large.

However, many cancerous tumors in the right colon commonly cause bleeding that is not visible in the stool. The blood
loss can be serious enough to lead to loss of iron, severe iron-deficiency anemia, and a general feeling of weakness or fatigue. In
very severe cases, anemia can lead to other problems with the cir-
culation, such as:

- Congestive heart failure—inability of the heart to pump
  strongly enough to move the volume of fluid through the
  body;
- Angina—chest pain caused by loss of effective blood flow
  through the coronary arteries to the heart; or
- Claudication—cramping pains in the legs caused by lack of
  blood flow to the muscles.

Bleeding from cancers in the right colon tends to occur more slowly and at lower volume than bleeding from other sites. The blood may mix with the feces and be harder to notice. The fecal occult blood test (FOBT) described in Chapter 6 is important because it can accurately detect the presence of this hidden (occult) blood. In some cases, though, the bleeding is more extensive and more obvious. Moderate or severe bleeding causes stools to appear deep red or maroon in color.

About 13 percent of colorectal cancers develop in the cecum, and another 9 percent develop in the right colon. For reasons we do not yet understand, although the overall rate of colorectal cancer is declining in the United States, the rate of tumors that develop in the right colon is on the rise. Early reports have suggested that this increase affects especially African American men. Perhaps better medical technology and greater public awareness of the disease have simply led to a higher chance that cancer will be diagnosed in this region. It may also be true that diet or some other factor is causing more tumors to develop in this part of the body.

The colon becomes narrower and less flexible as it progresses toward the rectum. The fecal matter also becomes drier and firmer. Cancers of the left colon and sigmoid colon are more likely to grow and form a complete ring around the colon, creating what doctors sometimes call a "napkin ring" effect. For these reasons, tumors that develop in the transverse colon (the horizontal section) or especially the left (descending) and sigmoid colon are more likely to lead to blockage. These cancers also tend to penetrate more deeply into the lining of the intestine, which can lead to visible bleeding.

Obstruction is a main cause of changes of bowel habit due to colorectal cancer. Constipation—the inability to have a regular bowel movement—results when the colon narrows and blocks the passage of feces. However, some people with colon cancer may develop the opposite problem—diarrhea—if contractions of the bowel force feces past a cancer that partially blocks the organ. This is sometimes known as "paradoxical diarrhea."

Abdominal pain can arise when a tumor causes the colon to stretch and press against nerves or other nearby tissues. The cramping is often worse after meals because eating triggers the rhythmic bowel contractions known as peristalsis. Some people who suffer from cramps mistakenly take laxatives for relief. (Cramping can also be caused by excess use of laxatives.)

Cancers in the rectum often cause bleeding, obstruction, and diarrhea. Rectal cancers typically cause tenesmus—increased straining due to a feeling that the bowel has not been completely emptied during a movement. Other symptoms of rectal cancer include increased frequency of stools; changes in stool consistency and diameter; small amounts of bright red bleeding; sudden and overwhelming urges to have a bowel movement (fecal urgency), and inability to control defecation (fecal incontinence).

As the cancer grows and spreads, the pattern of symptoms changes. Advanced cancers—those that penetrate into the layers of the intestine or into other nearby tissues—can cause pain in the region around the anus. They can also produce blood in the urine, increased urination (urinary frequency), and an abnormal channel (known as a fistula) between the colon or rectum and another organ, such as the vagina. If the tumor penetrates through the outer wall of the colon, fecal material may leak into the abdominal cavity, causing infection and fever and pain. Loss of appetite and weight loss are frequent signs of advanced cancer. Weakness and a general feeling of poor health (malaise) can result from blood loss, but they can also result from the impact of cancer that has spread (metastasized) to other parts of the body.

Metastases from colorectal cancer can cause additional symptoms, depending on the site of the spread. If the tumor invades the membrane surrounding the abdomen (the peritoneum), pain in the back or abdomen may occur. As cancerous cells affect other parts of the abdomen, excess fluid (ascites) may build up between the layers of the peritoneum, causing swelling, discomfort, and difficulty in breathing. Similarly, if the cancer spreads to the spine or to bones in the pelvis, pain may be noticed in these regions.

Tumors growing outside the colon can press back into the intestine, resulting in bowel obstruction. Sometimes, the nerves and muscles can be damaged, causing the intestines to lose their ability to contract and push the feces along. The medical term for this problem is *ileus*. If the tumor has spread to the liver, pain in the upper right corner of the abdomen may be present. A doctor may also be able to feel a large mass in the liver. Jaundice—yellowing of the skin and the eyes, resulting from a buildup of bile—is a sign that the cancer has damaged the liver. Metastases in the lungs can lead to coughing and difficulty in breathing. As the cancer continues to advance, it usually leads to pronounced changes in eating habits, including loss of appetite with resultant weight loss.

In making a diagnosis, a doctor will make every effort to identify the real cause of a problem. Many of the symptoms of colorectal cancer are nonspecific—they can also be caused by a number of other conditions.

For example, bright red rectal bleeding can be due to harmless lesions such as hemorrhoids. It also may result from serious but noncancerous problems such as leaky intestinal blood vessels or inflammatory diseases such as colitis (an inflammatory bowel disease) or infection. Tenesmus, urgency, and diarrhea may also occur. In women, abdominal pain can arise from endometriosis, a condition in which tissue from the lining of the uterus breaks off and travels to other parts of the pelvic cavity. Diverticular disease—which causes sections of the inner lining of the intestine to protrude outward, forming little pockets—can cause bleeding as well as changes in bowel habits, such as constipation, cramping pain, and narrowed stool. If one of these diverticular pouches becomes perforated, an enclosed, infected, pus-filled area (called an abscess) may form.

Irritable bowel syndrome, a chronic disorder involving the nerves and muscles of the intestine, can involve alternating constipation and diarrhea, as well as pain in the left lower portion of the abdomen. Irritable bowel syndrome is the most common disorder of the intestine. In some instances, it is a lifelong condition. A pronounced change or worsening in the pattern of symptoms of irritable bowel syndrome may indicate that cancer is also present.

THE PROCESS OF DIAGNOSIS

In trying to figure out the nature of a problem, a doctor usually starts by taking a careful history. You will be asked a series of questions about your general health and your past medical problems, including whether any colon polyps have ever been diagnosed or removed. Questions about family members and their illnesses are particularly relevant because several forms of colorectal cancer can be inherited.

After the history, a physical examination is in order. To a trained observer, clues to various diseases can be seen in everything from the way a patient walks into the examining room to marks on his or her fingernails. Evidence of weight loss, jaundice, or paleness can trigger the suspicion that a serious disease is present.

During the exam, the doctor will feel the lymph nodes and various places in the abdomen, looking for enlargement of the liver, masses, nodules, or tenderness. Such signs can indicate that cancer is present. During a rectal examination, you may be asked to perform a Valsalva maneuver (holding your breath while bearing down, as if straining during a bowel movement). This action causes changes in the positions of the internal organs, sometimes bringing a tumor into a new position so that examiners can detect it with their fingers.

Usually, a nurse or assistant will collect samples of urine and blood to send to a laboratory for analysis. High levels of certain substances in the blood, such as urea or creatinine, suggest that the kidneys are not functioning properly. Sometimes, for example, rectal cancers can block the tubes carrying urine from the kidneys to the bladder (the ureters). A low level of iron usually indicates chronic blood loss, and a low albumin level in the blood suggests that something is wrong with the metabolism, usually involving the liver. Unusual amounts of enzymes produced by the liver and circulating in the blood also point to trouble in this important organ.

A blood test also can be done to measure the levels of a substance known as carcinoembryonic antigen (CEA). This protein is sometimes found in higher than normal amounts in people who have colorectal cancer, especially when the disease has spread to other sites in the body. Doctors who suspect the presence of the disease may do a blood test for CEA. It's important to understand, however, that not all doctors consider the CEA test to be a mandatory part of the diagnostic process. If you have early-stage colorectal cancer and are experiencing no symptoms, your CEA levels may be normal. The main value of this test comes later, as your doctors monitor your progress after surgery, during what we call the surveillance period. A rise in CEA level at that time is a clue that the cancer may have returned.

If screening tests for colorectal cancer—the digital rectal exam (DRE), fecal occult blood test (FOBT), flexible sigmoidoscopy, colonoscopy, or barium enemas—are positive, or if symptoms are present, further steps are needed to establish a diagnosis. The main tests used to diagnose colorectal cancer are the double contrast barium enema (DCBE) and the colonoscopy. I'll describe these in more detail shortly.

In the process of receiving a diagnosis of colorectal cancer, you will likely meet a number of physicians with different skills. The basic physical exam and screening tests are easily performed by a range of health care professionals, including family doctors and internists. Some of these care providers may also be qualified to perform a sigmoidoscopy, and they may offer that procedure in their offices or at neighboring clinics or hospitals. Often, though, the sigmoidoscopy and the colonoscopy are done by someone who specializes in using endoscopes, such as a gastroenterologist or a surgical endoscopist. The DCBE involves the use of X-rays and is handled by a radiologist. During diagnosis, you are likely to deal with various members of the medical staff, including nurses, physician's assistants, and technicians.

DOUBLE CONTRAST BARIUM ENEMA (DCBE)

To make a diagnosis of colorectal cancer, the doctor needs to look at the entire large intestine. Flexible sigmoidoscopy is a good method—as far as it goes. However, the scope used during this procedure can only look at 50 percent or less of the colon. To get a full survey of the terrain, physicians often supplement the sigmoidoscopy by administering a barium enema, sometimes called a double contrast enema, air contrast enema, or lower GI (gastrointestinal) series. Recent improvements in barium radiographic technology have made it possible for some patients to avoid having to undergo the sigmoidoscopic part of the exam.

During a DCBE, the colon is bathed in a milky substance (known as a medium) containing the element barium. The substance is administered through an enema, or a nozzle inserted into the rectum. After the medium has spread into the entire colon, an X-ray is taken. Because barium blocks X-rays, any abnormal growths or areas will show up on the film. This procedure offers physicians a way to get a picture of the entire colon. It is not a direct view, as can be obtained through a colonoscope, but it is useful for detecting cancers and large polyps and also for diagnosing the cause of any obstruction.

There are two types of barium enemas. The single contrast enema involves only the use of the barium medium and the X-ray. However, this method usually does not produce the most complete or accurate image possible. To enhance the quality, and to provide a more accurate diagnosis of colorectal cancer, many doctors prefer to use the double contrast barium enema

(DCBE). Most of the barium is removed and the colon is then inflated with air. This method, sometimes called an air contrast enema, expands the tissue. The special coating properties of the remaining barium make the contours of the organ—especially the smaller polyps or tumors—much easier to see in the X-ray image.

The DCBE is not painful or dangerous, but it does involve some discomfort and inconvenience. It is an outpatient procedure that takes about twenty to thirty minutes. Patients do not need to be anesthetized or sedated, but some doctors administer an intravenous drug that reduces the risk of muscle spasms. There is no need to be admitted to a hospital, but preparation for the DCBE begins twenty-four hours in advance. You will be asked to eat only a liquid diet, drink lots of clear fluids, and take laxatives and enemas. The goal is to wash as much material as possible out of the colon so that the X-ray will be clear and easy to read.

You will continue to pass the barium medium in your stool for up to two days after the procedure. Some people experience temporary constipation that may require use of laxatives. Temporary abdominal cramps arise afterward in perhaps one out of five patients.

DCBE is somewhat more complicated and expensive than the single contrast procedure, but it is much better at detecting cancerous or potentially cancerous lesions. Because it is a less intensive procedure, the single contrast enema is often administered to patients who are very young, very old, or seriously disabled. However, the single contrast enema misses about half of cancers and a majority of adenomas.

When used in combination with sigmoidoscopy, the DCBE is almost as good as colonoscopy for detecting lesions over 2 centimeters (cm) in size. The test will reveal between 50 and 80 percent of polyps less than 1 cm, 70 to 90 percent of polyps larger than 1 cm, and 55 to 80 percent of Stage I and II cancers. It is better at detecting cancer than the fecal occult blood test or sigmoidoscopy alone, because these tests cannot investigate the entire colon. DCBE is generally safer than sigmoidoscopy or colonoscopy because it does not involve insertion of a scope.

One main drawback of DCBE is that it can miss small polyps and adenomas; lesions that are less than 8 millimeters (mm) in diameter are difficult, if not impossible, to detect. About 5 to 10 percent of the images resulting from DCBE are not clear enough or complete enough to be of good diagnostic use. Also, X-ray images are just shadows of the internal organ. They can sometimes be difficult to read and interpret accurately. Bits of stool left inside the colon, or other noncancerous irregularities, can appear to be polyps or cancers; such findings are known as false positives. If the image is unclear, a colonoscopy will be required.

Another issue to be aware of is that the barium enema does not allow the physician to remove or biopsy any polyps or cancerous tumors that might turn up during the procedure. Consequently, patients who have abnormal results on DCBE will still have to undergo a colonoscopy.

The most serious risks from DCBE are bowel perforation, which occurs in 1 out of 25,000 cases, and cardiac complications, which affect 1 in 46,000 patients. The amount of radiation a patient is exposed to during a procedure is not large—300 to 500 millirems. (For comparison, a standard mammogram involves exposure to 300 millirems.)

For what it's worth, surveys find that between 50 and 94 percent of patients undergoing a DCBE rate the procedure as "acceptable"—in other words, it is no one's idea of the most pleasant way to spend a morning, but it could be worse.

COLONOSCOPY

The best diagnostic tool currently available for identifying colorectal cancer is the colonoscope. This tool is typically used for a follow-up examination if other screening or diagnostic tests produce positive results. If a lesion is found by sigmoidoscopy or DCBE, colonoscopy gives doctors a close-up look so they can ascertain the nature of the tissue, remove it if it is a benign-appearing adenoma, obtain a tissue sample if it is a malignant lesion, and make certain there are no other lesions growing at the same time farther up in the colon. About 50 percent of patients whose FOBT indicates bleeding for the first time will be found, during a colonoscopy, to have a suspicious lesion; about 38 percent of these lesions will be adenomas (potential cancers) and 12 percent will be carcinomas (cancerous tumors). Colonoscopy is also the main diagnostic procedure for individuals at high risk for colorectal cancer. Some experts recommend that people undergo screening with colonoscopy every ten years.

One key advantage of colonoscopy is that the scope is 150 cm (60 inches, or 5 feet) long, so it can be used to examine the entire large intestine. The device is designed to allow a polypectomy (a procedure in which the doctor snips off polyps) or the removal of samples of suspicious-looking tissue.

Preparation for the procedure involves the same steps as for the DCBE: a special liquid diet and a thorough bowel cleansing. This can be done with laxatives, but it also usually involves enemas or swallowing large amounts (nearly a gallon) of a nonabsorbable solution that contains various salts and triggers bowel movements.

You need to be awake during a colonoscopy, because you must be able to respond to instructions or tell the doctor doing the procedure whether you feel any pain or discomfort. You will probably receive a drug to provide some degree of sedation, but anesthesia is not needed. As in the DCBE, air is introduced through the endoscope to inflate the intestine and make it easier to examine.

The physician (usually a gastroenterologist or an endoscopist) maneuvers the scope within the bowel and watches the progress through a lens or on a video monitor (Figure 7.1). Any polyps detected can be removed with a device that uses electricity and heat and looks like a tiny wire lasso (Figure 7.2). The procedure takes at least fifteen to forty-five minutes; the actual time depends on the

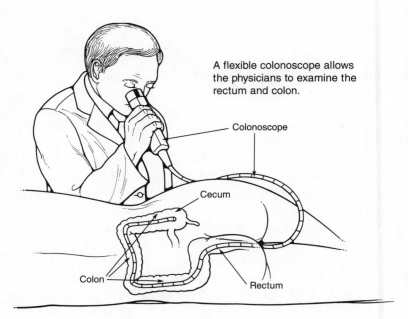

A flexible colonoscope allows the physicians to examine the rectum and colon.

Colonoscope

Cecum

Colon

Rectum

Figure 7.1: Colonoscopy.

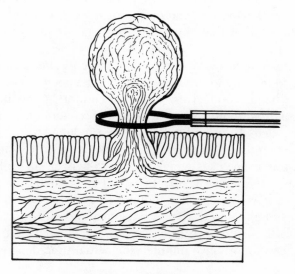

Figure 7.2: Polypectomy.

experience of the physician and the type and extent of lesions detected. Afterward, you will be taken to a recovery room to rest for an hour or two while the sedation wears off. In surveys of patient acceptability, colonoscopy and DCBE are rated about the same.

The colonoscope is able to examine the entire colon, from the rectum to the cecum, in about 95 percent of procedures. If, for some reason, the whole colon cannot be seen—due to obstruction or some other complication—the procedure is brought to an end. In such cases, either a DCBE or a repeat colonoscopy may be needed at a later time.

The procedure is effective in detecting both polyps and cancers. Understandably, the smaller the polyp, the less accurate the detection. Studies have found that colonoscopy misses up to 25 percent of polyps less than 5 mm in diameter and 10 percent of polyps greater than 1 cm.

Some risks are involved, especially if polyp removal is done during the procedure. The major complications are perforation of the bowel (occurring in 1 case out of 1,000), serious bleeding (3 cases per 1,000), and respiratory problems due to sedation (5 cases per 1,000). Abnormal heart rhythms, infection, and pain (during and after the procedure) can occur. The risk of death from the procedure is between 1 and 3 out of 10,000.

THE ISSUE OF STAGING

Identifying that cancer is present is only one part of the diagnosis. The other is to determine what stage the cancer has reached. The stages of colorectal cancer are described in Appendix 1. As discussed in Chapter 3, the earlier the stage at diagnosis, the more hopeful the possible outcomes of treatment.

Your physicians will collect and analyze all the available clues to determine the stage of your cancer prior to treatment. This is known as clinical staging. You might be asked to have X-rays, or, in some cases, CT ("CAT") scans of your lungs or liver to determine whether the cancer has metastasized.

Additional diagnostic and staging tests are often given to people with rectal cancer because these tumors are closer to the body surface and can be seen more easily with special instruments. For example, endorectal ultrasound involves use of a probe inserted into the rectum. The probe emits sound waves that bounce off the tissues inside the body. The waves create a shadow image on a viewing scope that is similar to an X-ray but does not involve the use of radiation. This method can reveal how deeply a tumor has penetrated and whether nearby lymph nodes are involved. Doctors use this information to plan an operation or radiation therapy. Similarly, some patients with rectal cancer undergo pelvic scans with CT or another technology called magnetic resonance imaging (MRI).

After the suspicious lesions have been removed—whether through biopsy or surgery—they, along with any lymph nodes removed at the same time, will be studied under a microscope. A pathologist who examines the tissues under a microscope will then determine the actual stage of the cancer. This more accurate assessment is known as pathological staging.

SECOND OPINIONS

Receiving a diagnosis of cancer and making choices about treatments can be a difficult and upsetting process. Fortunately, in most cases of colorectal cancer, you have time to consider your options carefully before taking any action. (The exception is if the cancer is causing serious bleeding or is blocking the intestine. Emergency surgery may then be needed.)

It is a good idea to get a second opinion before agreeing to any form of treatment for colorectal cancer. Seeing another physician serves several purposes. You may learn about other treatment possibilities, including innovative new approaches. If both doctors agree on a treatment strategy, you will feel more confident that the choice is right for you. Many insurance companies require (and will reimburse for) a second opinion concerning a major procedure such as cancer surgery.

Don't worry about how your doctor will react if you or members of your family suggest getting a second opinion. Good doctors know that patients wrestling with tough decisions about cancer need all the support and information they can obtain. Your doctor should be able to refer you to other physicians who will review your situation and make suggestions. Feel free to discuss each doctor's opinion with the other. Doing so will help raise your level of confidence that the choice you ultimately make is the right one for you.

Chapter 8

Surgery

Treatment is available for every person with cancer of the colon, rectum, or anus, regardless of what stage the cancer has reached. The three main approaches to treatment are:

1. Surgery—an operation to remove the tumor and affected nearby tissues, including lymph nodes, from the body.
2. Radiation—use of high-energy rays to penetrate the body and kill the cancer cells.
3. Chemotherapy—use of cancer-killing drugs that circulate in the body.

In the near future, biological therapies may also play an important role. These include immunotherapy, manipulation of the body's own immune system. Additional biological therapies aim to influence the way cancer cells signal each other, or to interfere with the proteins called growth factors that stimulate growth of cancer cells.

Often, treatment for colorectal cancer involves a combination of these methods. For that reason, you will likely receive medical attention from a number of physicians who have expertise in different fields. This is known as a multidisciplinary approach. The types of physicians involved in treating colorectal cancer include surgeons, radiation oncologists, and medical oncologists (specialists in cancer treatment). They in turn will consult diagnostic radiologists and pathologists, who will provide other important information. Depending on your individual needs, your team might also include nurses, social workers, stoma therapists, and others.

At times, it may be confusing to deal with so many different medical specialists and supportive care personnel. Keep in mind, however, that having a team of experts involved in your care gives you the best chance of receiving the most complete and advanced treatment available. Today, the multidisciplinary approach is practiced at the leading comprehensive cancer care centers throughout the country.

The main treatment for colon cancer, and the focus of this chapter, is surgery. In many cases, this may be the only approach needed. When performed for early-stage colon cancer, surgery alone achieves a complete cure in three out of four cases.

Depending on the location and type of tumor, however, a combination of treatment methods may be needed. Advanced colon cancer usually involves use of drugs in addition to surgery. Rectal cancer often responds to a combination of surgery and radiation, and all but the most superficial anal cancers are treated using chemotherapy and radiation. The therapeutic options depend very much on the stage of the cancer at the time of diagnosis. The more advanced the disease, the more complex the therapy will be. Tables 8.1 and 8.2 summarize these options. (For more information about staging, see Appendix 1.)

In some cases, drugs or radiation may be given before a surgical operation in an effort to shrink the tumor and make it easier to remove, or they may be used during the operation to reduce the risk that cancerous cells may spread to other tissues. Use of additional treatment prior to or during the main form of treatment is known as *neoadjuvant therapy*.

In other cases, drugs or radiation (or both) may be administered after surgery to destroy any cells that may have been left behind or that may have already spread to other sites in the body. This method is called *adjuvant therapy*. Chapter 9 describes in more detail the nonsurgical approaches, including the use of drugs

TABLE 8.1: TREATMENT OPTIONS FOR COLORECTAL CANCER

Stage	Description	Surgical Strategy
Stage 0	Malignant polyp (sometimes called carcinoma in situ)—cancerous cells do not penetrate beyond the tip of the polyp	Polypectomy of local excision
Stage I	Tumor remains within bowel wall	Surgical removal of part of colon
Stage II	Tumor penetrates through the bowel wall	Surgical removal of part of colon Possible clinical trials
Stage III	Cancerous cells found in nearby lymph nodes	Surgical removal of part of colon Chemotherapy Clinical trials
Stage IV	Cancer has spread to other sites	Surgical removal of part of colon Surgical removal of other affected tissue (for example, liver) Chemotherapy Radiation Clinical trials
Recurrent	Cancer has returned despite treatment	Possible repeat colon surgery Surgery to remove metastases Palliative chemotherapy Palliative radiation Clinical trials

under study in experiments known as *clinical trials* or *protocols*. In Chapter 12, I'll describe additional steps for dealing with recurrent cancer—disease that returns despite an aggressive course of treatment.

SURGERY FOR CANCER OF THE LARGE INTESTINE

As noted above, surgery is the most common treatment for colon cancer. If the cancer is not large or it does not penetrate very far, all that may be needed is a polypectomy (removal of the polyp) or a local excision (removal of a small amount of tissue from the inner surface of the intestine or the skin of the anus).

TABLE 8.2: TREATMENT OPTIONS FOR ANAL CANCER		
Stage	**Description**	**Surgical Strategy**
Stage 0	Small tumors on the anal skin or in the anal canal	Local excision
Stage I	Tumors less than 2 cm on the skin or in the anal canal	Radiation Chemotherapy Surgery (if response to other treatments is incomplete)
Stage II	Tumors larger than 2 cm	Radiation Chemotherapy Surgery (if response to other treatments is incomplete)
Stage IIIA	Cancer involves rectal lymph nodes or nearby organs	Radiation Surgery Chemotherapy Clinical trials
Stage IIIB	Cancer involves other pelvic lymph nodes	Radiation Chemotherapy Surgery Clinical trials
Stage IV	Cancer has spread to other sites	Palliative surgery Palliative radiation Palliative chemotherapy Clinical trials
Recurrent		Surgery Radiation Chemotherapy Clinical trials

More extensive cancers require surgery (also called *resection)* to completely remove part or all of the colon, along with any lymph nodes and nearby blood vessels that might contain cancerous cells. An operation performed in hopes of eradicating the cancer is called *curative surgery.* (Types of cancer-related surgery are defined in the box on page 122.)

The earlier surgery is done, the better the chances of a cure. If the disease remains localized—that is, it has not spread to other tissues or organs—resection will result in a cure about 75 percent of the time. The overall cure rate, which includes surgery performed for colorectal cancer at all stages, is about 50 percent. Even if the cancer has metastasized to a single spot on the liver, surgery (including surgery to remove the affected portion of the liver) may produce a cure in about 20 percent of patients. Surgery accounts for more cures in large bowel cancer than all other forms of treatment combined.

Almost all colorectal cancers can be treated with surgery. Sometimes, though, doctors decide that a tumor is too large or involves too much neighboring tissue to be removed safely. In such cases, a course of radiation or chemotherapy may be given before the operation to cause the tumor to shrink in size. Cancer that has spread into other tissues may actually retreat from those places after exposure to drugs or radiation. If this retreat occurs, the surgery performed has an excellent chance of providing good results.

Generally, once colorectal cancer has been diagnosed, there is no need to rush into surgery. The disease may have been developing for years. If you learn that you have colorectal cancer, try to remain calm. You are not in immediate danger. You have time to talk with your doctors about the best options available to you, to make plans for your stay in the hospital, to get a second opinion, and so on. The exception is when a tumor is bleeding or causing bowel obstruction. Emergency surgery may then be needed.

Even if a cure is not possible, surgery can still provide benefit by relieving problems associated with the disease, such as bleeding or intestinal blockage. Surgery undertaken to improve the situation or relieve symptoms is known as *palliative surgery*.

Whenever possible following resection, the surgeon will try to reconnect the intestine so that it can continue to function. Doing so avoids the need for a permanent or temporary *colostomy*, an opening in the abdominal wall through which feces can pass out of the body. When most people face decisions about their treatment, fear of a colostomy is often among their greatest concerns. Fortunately, when modern surgical techniques are used, the rate of permanent colostomy following colon surgery is only about 3 percent or less. I'll have more to say about colostomies later in this chapter.

The surgery for rectal cancer is somewhat different than for colon cancer. Depending on the extent of the cancer, polypectomy, local excision, local resection, or electrosurgery may be performed. These methods do not require "open" surgery (an incision in the abdomen). Instead, they can be done using instruments inserted through the anus.

However, if the rectal cancer is more extensive, part of the rectum must be removed. Stage I, II, or III rectal cancer usually requires either low anterior (LA) resection or abdominoperineal (AP) resection.

LA resection is used for cancers near the upper part of the rectum, close to where it connects with the colon. After LA resection, the colon is attached to the anus and waste is eliminated in the usual way.

AP resection is used for cancer in the lower part of the rectum, close to its outer connection to the anus. After AP resection, a colostomy is needed.

A *pelvic exenteration* is a procedure done if the cancer has spread to nearby organs. In this surgery, the rectum as well as nearby organs, such as the bladder, prostate (in men), or uterus (in women), are removed. Colostomy is needed after a pelvic exenteration.

In anal cancer, surgery produces a cure in about 50 percent of cases. The problem is that an operation in this region often affects the *sphincter*, a ring of muscles in the anus that controls the passage of feces. Damage to or loss of the sphincter means a permanent colostomy will be needed. For this reason, radiation and chemotherapy are the treatments of choice for cancer of the anus. These approaches result in five-year survival rates of 75 percent.

THE PROCESS OF SURGERY

Surgery for colorectal cancer is a major operation that will require hospitalization. Depending on your condition, you may not need to be admitted to the hospital until the day of the procedure.

TYPES OF CANCER SURGERY

Cryosurgery destroys tumors by freezing them and is most successful if tumors are easily seen or felt. Cryosurgery is usually performed on cancers of the head, neck, liver, and skin.

Definitive or *curative* surgery is the removal of a tumor and adjacent lymph nodes when the tumor appears to be localized and there is hope of taking out all of the cancerous tissue.

Diagnostic surgery is a tissue biopsy to confirm a diagnosis or identify the specific cancer.

Electrosurgery (also called *electrofulguration),* the use of high-frequency current, is done for some cancers of the skin, mouth, colon, and rectum.

Laser surgery is performed using a laser beam, which is a concentrated ray of high-energy light.

Local excision removes superficial cancers and a small amount of nearby tissue.

Local full thickness resection involves cutting through all layers of the rectum to remove invasive cancers as well as some surrounding tissue.

Palliative surgery is performed as a treatment of complications of advanced disease and is done to relieve pain. It is also performed in an effort to stem spread of the disease.

Preventive surgery is performed to remove a growth not presently malignant, when the surgeon feels it might become malignant if left untreated. This type of surgery is used for precancerous conditions such as polyps in the colon and moles on the skin. People with hereditary syndromes who are at high risk of developing colorectal cancer usually undergo preventive surgery to remove the colon or rectum (or both).

Radical surgery is the removal of the tumor and lymph glands in addition to any adjacent tissues or organs affected by cancer cells, such as nerves, muscles, or blood vessels.

Staging surgery is done not to treat the disease but to determine how extensive it is. This determination may also be accomplished by laparoscopy (see pages 133–134).

One or two days before the operation, however, you will need to undergo a thorough bowel cleansing. This step is important for a successful outcome, because it removes all the contents from the intestine and reduces the number of bacteria present. Typically, you will be asked to drink about a gallon of a special liquid that acts to flush out the bowel. Alternately, doctors will recommend a three-day regimen involving enemas and doses of a laxative called magnesium citrate. You will remain on a clear liquid diet during this preparation.

To further reduce risk of infection, you will be asked to take oral antibiotics (such as erythromycin and neomycin) on the day prior to surgery. During and after the operation, you will receive intravenous antibiotics to help protect the surgical sites against infection. These antibiotics are called "broad-spectrum" because they kill a wide range of potentially harmful bacteria.

You will be given an anesthetic to make you unconscious and free of pain. Before the operation, you will meet the anesthesiologist, who will explain what will be done and make sure you are not allergic to any of the drugs used to produce anesthesia.

The procedure takes approximately two to four hours, depending on such factors as how much body fat there is and how much tissue must be removed. Even the most extensive diagnostic testing done beforehand may not reveal everything that is going on inside your body. Surgeons may not know exactly what they need to do during the operation until they can actually see the tissue involved. If, for example, the tumor is more extensive than was believed, the operation can take longer, or additional procedures may be needed.

After the procedure, you will be taken to a recovery room where nurses and other medical personnel will keep an eye on you as the anesthesia wears off. You will probably remain in the hospital for three to six days while your body heals. Antibiotics will be administered intravenously to prevent infection. Once normal bowel sounds return—usually within a day or so—you will be able to eat again. Usually, during your stay, your surgeon and a stoma therapist will teach you how to take care of your colostomy (if you have one).

Once back home, you should plan to rest completely. Avoid lifting or moving heavy objects. About a week after the procedure, you will be asked to return to the hospital or outpatient office so your doctor can remove your stitches and examine the surgical site to make sure all is well.

For a period of time—weeks, or perhaps months—you may experience more frequent bowel movements and your stool may be watery. However, in most cases, the bowel patterns return to normal after a while.

PARTS OF THE COLON OR RECTUM REMOVED DURING SURGERY

You may wonder why large sections of the colon, or the entire colon, must be removed during surgery for cancer, when the tumor may only directly affect a relatively small area of tissue. The answer has to do with the nature of the disease and its ability to spread and metastasize. Cancers can penetrate into the lymphatic vessels and blood vessels that run through the wall of the intestine. Cutting into these vessels can dislodge cancerous cells and might increase the risk that they will travel elsewhere in the body and grow as metastases. To prevent this, surgeons make their incisions at sites located some distance from the affected areas.

Similarly, cancers can penetrate the bowel wall and involve the network of vessels (called the mesentery) that nourishes those sections of tissue. Spread of cancer usually follows a predictable route. Consequently, surgeons must be careful to remove entire sections of the colon as well as the vessels and lymph nodes associated with those sections that are most likely to be involved. This approach is somewhat like the strategy of law enforcement officials who seal off major streets to trap a thief who is trying to escape via the fastest route out of town.

Another reason is that, for surgery to produce a cure, all affected tissue must be taken out. The goal is to achieve what surgeons call negative (or "clean") margins. This term means that the edges of tissue removed, when studied under a microscope, prove to have no cancerous cells in them. That's what surgeons mean when they say, "We got it all."

The anatomy of the large bowel is basically the same in every human being. For this reason, surgeons use certain defined boundaries to identify the sections that must be removed. The extent of the operation (shown by doted lines) illustrated in Figure 8.1 may vary somewhat based on the cancer's exact location within each bowel region.

- A *right radical hemicolectomy* (Figure 8.1A) is performed to remove tumors that affect the cecum and the ascending colon (shaded area). This operation removes essentially half of the colon (*hemi-* means "half"), including the cecum, the ascending colon, the hepatic flexure (the "corner" where the ascending colon makes a 90-degree turn), and the first third of the transverse colon (the area outlined with a dotted line). An *extended right hemicolectomy* removes more and is used for cancers of the hepatic flexure of the transverse colon.
- A *transverse colectomy*, performed to treat cancers of the transverse colon, involves removal of the horizontal part of the colon, including the two "corners" (the hepatic and the splenic flexures).
- A *left radical hemicolectomy* (Figure 8.1B) is performed when the tumor resides in the descending colon or the splenic fixture. The extent of surgery varies somewhat according to the exact location of the tumor. For cancers of the splenic flexure this operation removes about a third of the transverse colon, the splenic flexure, and the first half of the descending colon. A left hemicolectomy for a descending colon tumor will remove the descending colon and splenic flexure (the area within the dotted line).

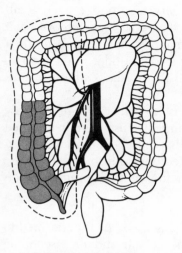

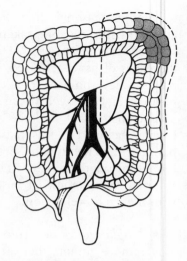

A. Right radical hemicolectomy

B. Left radical hemicolectomy

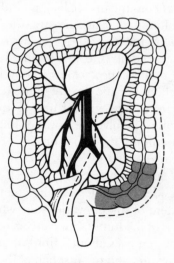

C. Sigmoid resection

Figure 8.1: Types of colectomy.

- A *sigmoid resection*, (Figure 8.1C) is indicated when the tumor affects the sigmoid section of the colon (shaded area). It involves removal of about two-thirds of the descending colon and all of the sigmoid colon (as outlined with a dotted line). The surgeon will leave intact as much of the rectum as possible.

- A *rectosigmoid resection* includes all of the sigmoid colon and much or all of the rectum and tissue next to the rectum (the mesorectum). Depending on the extent of cancerous tissue, the surgeon will meticulously strive to leave intact the tissue where the rectum and the anus meet. Doing so reduces the risk that a permanent colostomy will be needed.

- *Abdominoperineal resection* is the procedure for treating some rectal cancers that have penetrated into the intestinal wall. This operation often involves removal of the sphincter and poses the greatest need for permanent colostomy. It is usually done only in patients with cancer that affects the lower third of the rectum and has penetrated to the muscle layer of the intestine.

- *Transanal* or *transsphincteric resection* refers to surgery designed to remove small superficial cancers in the rectum. This operation can be done using instruments inserted through the anal opening, rather than through a surgical incision in the abdomen.

- *Low anterior resection* is used for cancers of the upper or middle thirds of the rectum. This operation removes tissue from the lower half of the sigmoid colon to 3 cm (about 1 inch) below the location of the rectal cancer.

After making the incision and examining the abdomen, surgeons may see that the tumor also affects adjacent organs, especially the urinary organs and, in women, the reproductive organs, including the ovaries. This is the case in about 10 percent of large bowel cancers, especially those arising in the rectum and the rectosigmoid colon. These tumors may be limited to the outer surface of the other organs, or they may actually invade these tissues. In most of these instances, the surgeon will go ahead and remove as much of the affected tissue as possible. Such a step is necessary to achieve negative margins and provide the best chance of a cure.

Also, during the operation, the surgeon may discover that the colorectal cancer has metastasized to the liver. This happens in 20 to 25 percent of cases. (Use of ultrasound during abdominal surgery may increase the ability of the surgeon to detect these metastases.) If only one metastatic site is involved and it is small, the affected tissue can be removed while you are undergoing surgery for the primary tumor in the colon. Often, though, you may need to have another operation six or eight weeks later to re-move liver tumors, particularly if more than one is found. You will also need to undergo additional imaging tests so your doctors can pinpoint the exact size and location of the liver tumors before that operation. Research shows that surgery to remove metastatic liver tumors may increase, by perhaps 40 percent, the chances of surviving five years or more.

PALLIATIVE SURGERY

Prior to surgery, your doctors will do all they can to correctly de-termine the stage of your cancer. Even so, the most accurate stag-ing can only be done at the time of the procedure. This is known as intraoperative staging. Sometimes, the cancer turns out to be more advanced than was previously known. For this reason, some treatment decisions can only be made when the operation is in progress.

Even if the colorectal cancer has metastasized, surgeons will almost always try to remove the original tumor. This approach will not result in a cure, but it is palliative—that is, it can lessen the chance of problems down the road. In rare cases of ad-vanced disease, such as when risk of further spread is high or part of the small intestine is affected, the surgeons may decide not to remove the affected area. In such cases, the choice is to perform an intestinal bypass, attaching the colon to create a "detour" around the tumor.

Large, bulky rectal tumors will be removed despite the presence of metastatic disease. Often, though, you may need preoperative radiation or chemotherapy, or both, to reduce the size of the tumor and make the surgery less hazardous. Removing tumors reduces the risk of persistent pelvic problems such as tenesmus (painful urge to have a bowel movement), rectal or anal pain, loss of mucus, burning, and bleeding, and greatly reduces the suffering that rectal cancer can cause. If possible, the surgeons will try to save the sphincter and avoid a colostomy. However, if the risk is high that the cancer will recur, a colostomy is the better option in the long run, because it can add years to one's life.

When the tumor in the lower rectum is small, the doctors may recommend a series of procedures in which the cancerous cells are destroyed by an electrical probe or by a special form of radiation therapy. This increases the number of visits to the physician over the years to come, but some people would prefer that to having a permanent colostomy.

LAPAROSCOPY

The standard colorectal cancer operation is known as *open surgery*, because an incision is made in the abdomen and the skin is opened. This permits a good view of the area and good access for the doctors and their surgical tools.

Recent developments in medical technology have led to the creation of smaller and smaller instruments known as laparoscopes. Because these devices are of such small diameter, they can be inserted through slits in the skin that are only about one-half inch long. Gas is gently pumped into the opening area to expand the tissue. Then tiny video cameras with lights on the end are inserted through the slits. The cameras are attached to viewing monitors and can be manipulated to give the surgeon—and everyone else in the operating room—a bright, clear view of the area being treated. Small surgical tools inserted through other openings can then be used to perform the procedure. After the work is done, the gas is released and the slits are sewn together with sutures.

During the past few years, laparoscopic surgery has revolutionized the treatment of many medical conditions, including gall bladder disease and gynecologic disorders. A similar instrument, the arthroscope, is used in joint surgery. Some physicians are now using laparoscopic surgery to treat colorectal cancer. In theory, the advantages of laparoscopy include smaller incisions, less trauma to the colon and the abdomen, less risk of pain or infection, faster recovery times, and shorter hospital stays.

However, at this time, we simply don't have enough evidence to state with certainty that this approach is as safe and effective as traditional open surgery. As explained earlier, one problem with colorectal cancer treatment is that the surgeon often needs to directly view a large portion of the abdominal cavity to know how extensive the disease is. Using a tiny scope that can show only a small area at a time may increase the risk of missing signs that the cancer has spread or that other organs and tissues are involved. Another concern is that effective colorectal cancer surgery requires removal of the lymph nodes. Evidence is not yet available showing that nodes can be removed completely and effectively when using laparoscopic methods.

There are other concerns. Laparoscopy actually takes longer than conventional surgery, at least until the surgeon has performed several dozen such operations. Nor is it necessarily cheaper, because of the additional equipment involved and the need for highly trained specialists and treatment facilities. One recent study found that laparoscopy offered no advantage over conventional methods in terms of postoperative complications, use of anesthesia, or the speed with which the bowel returned to its normal function. Further, there is the chance that tumor cells may implant and grow at the site of instrument placement through the abdominal wall. Because the technology is new, we do not yet have the results of long-term studies showing whether laparoscopy offers advantages in terms of survival and improved quality of life. It will be five years or more before such results are available.

The method shows some promise, but it is still in its infancy and cannot be recommended—yet—as the "gold standard" of care. Studies are under way that will help us resolve these questions; for example, a major study is being sponsored by the National Cancer Institute. Until we know more, some experts advise against using laparoscopy-assisted colectomy as a substitute for conventional open surgery unless the surgeon performing the procedure is specially trained in, and committed to using, this technique.

POTENTIAL COMPLICATIONS OF COLORECTAL SURGERY

After removing the section of colon, the surgeon uses sutures or staples to attach the two severed ends to each other. This process is called *reconstruction*; the resulting connection is known as an *anastomosis* (Figure 8.2). During the healing process, the rejoined tissues eventually fuse back together. However, the connection might not be entirely secure, especially during the early phases of recovery, and fecal material can seep out of the connection and into the abdominal cavity. The result can be infection, inflammation, and other potentially serious complications. The risk of problems caused by an insecure anastomosis depends on various factors, including the skill of the surgeon and the amount of "pulling" between the two rejoined sections of the intestine. In some cases, modern stapling devices appear to produce better results than sewing by hand.

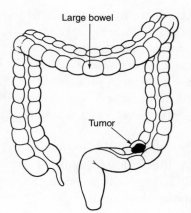
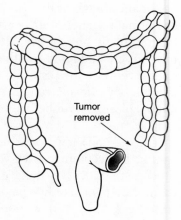
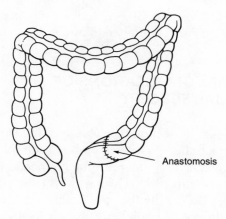

Figure 8.2: Anastomosis.

Cancers in the rectosigmoid colon are sometimes trickier to operate on than tumors in other parts of the bowel. Tumors in this region tend to involve other organs, including the bladder or, in women, the uterus. Additional steps may be needed during the operation. For example, catheters may need to be introduced to allow urine to drain away and to make the site of the operation easier for the surgeon to see.

The nerves that trigger erections in men are located near the rectum. There is a significant chance that surgery for colorectal cancer, especially for rectal cancer, can damage or destroy these nerves. Sometimes, too, the cancer has spread to these tissues and they have to be removed. As a consequence, after the operation, some men experience impotence (erectile dysfunction), defined as an inability to achieve and sustain an erection sufficient for sexual intercourse. The risk that men will experience sexual problems after colorectal surgery depends on how extensively the operation removed the rectum and nearby tissues, as well as the patient's age at the time of surgery. Older men were more susceptible to this side effect. Impotence occurred in nearly half of men undergoing abdomino perineal resection and about 15 percent of those having low anterior resection. In women, damage to nerves in this region can lead to problems with the bladder and loss of urinary control. Some women may also lose their ability to experience orgasm.

The good news is that, in recent years, doctors have developed ways of performing colorectal surgery that offer a greater chance of preserving these nerves. Among the many factors that determine whether this method can be used are: the distance of the cancer from the boundary between the anus and the rectum; the size and type of tumor; the involvement of adjacent organs and tissues in the cancer; and the width of the pelvis.

Naturally, an operation as complex as colorectal cancer surgery poses a risk of bleeding. Modern techniques reduce this danger considerably, but some patients will need to undergo blood transfusions during the course of the procedure. It is the practice in some hospitals to suggest that patients donate their own blood prior to an operation. Autologous transfusions (transfusions of one's own blood) pose less of a risk of infection or other complications than blood from unknown donors (allogenic transfusions). If you are concerned about this issue, talk it over with the members of your cancer care team.

During an operation, doctors take exquisite care to make sure no cancerous cells break free and escape into the abdominal cavity. Precautionary steps include use of special materials to isolate the surgical site, or use of saline fluid to bathe the area at the end of the operation.

Infection is always a risk following surgery. Antibiotics are given before, during, and after, to reduce the chances of infection.

A WORD ABOUT COLOSTOMY

For most people with colorectal cancer, the possibility of having a colostomy after surgery is a source of great concern. As noted earlier, a colostomy is a surgically created opening between the bowel and the abdominal wall. Through this opening, feces pass out of the body and into a collection bag.

There are different types of ostomies, depending on the site of the cancer and the operation performed. For example, an ileostomy may be needed if the entire colon and rectum has been removed. In this case, the opening extends from the ileum, the lowest portion of the small intestine. Removal of the entire colon and rectum is rarely needed to treat colon or rectal cancer. Exceptions include treatment of patients with more than one primary cancer in the colon and the rectum, and preventive removal of the colon and rectum in some patients with very strong colorectal cancer risk factors.

In the vast majority of cases, the colon can be reconnected in patients with adequately prepared bowel, and no colostomy will be created. The risk rises if surgery has to be performed on an emergency basis, as when the bowel is obstructed or perforated (temporary colostomy). Colostomies are also usually required after surgery of the lower rectum, in which the sphincter muscles must be destroyed because of the overriding need to eradicate every bit of cancerous tissue.

Overall, only about 3 percent of patients undergoing colorectal cancer surgery will need to have a permanent colostomy. A larger percentage of patients will require a temporary colostomy. After the bowel has been allowed to heal for a while, another operation can be performed to remove and rejoin the remaining bowel. The time for healing varies; in most cases, it is two or three months, but it can be as short as a few weeks or as long as a year or more.

When discussing treatment options with your caregivers, you will be told in advance about the potential need for a colostomy in your case. Don't hesitate to voice any concerns you have. Your medical team will probably include a person who is specially trained in this area. This person, sometimes called a stoma therapist, can answer any questions you might have. If an ostomy is necessary after your operation, this person will mark your skin at the best site for the colostomy and will be available to teach you how to manage your colostomy: keeping it clean, changing the collection bag, taking care of the skin, and so on. Some therapists will make home visits.

Most people who have a colostomy can lead fully normal and productive lives. Sometimes the biggest problem with a colostomy involves dealing with family, friends, or coworkers who do not understand your situation. The therapist can help by providing education and support. Patient groups such as the United Ostomy Association provide information and guidance. The American Cancer Society offers booklets and other materials. For more information, see Chapter 12 and the Resources section at the end of this book.

COPING WITH A COLOSTOMY:
ONE MAN'S STORY

"When the doctor explained that I would need to have part of my colon removed, he also told me that I would probably end up with a sigmoid colostomy," recalled Jack, a 54-year-old construction contractor. "The whole idea scared me so much that I kind of shut down and didn't really listen. I remember thinking, 'If I have to go through the rest of my life crapping into a bag attached to my body, my life is pretty much over.' I couldn't travel, I couldn't work out at the gym, I wouldn't dream of going golfing with my buddies or going to parties. What if I was giving off odor, or what if the bag got loose and I made a mess of myself?

"And I thought, 'Well, that's the end of my sex life, too.' I mean, my wife Rachel's a good woman. I love her dearly and she's pretty understanding. But she's no saint, and you'd have to be a saint to forget that the person you're making love with has this . . . this hole in the side of his body. I wondered if she'd want to leave me, and then I tried to imagine dating again. No way.

"Finding out I had cancer was bad enough. But the more I learned about the colostomy, the more I felt that the cure might be worse than the disease. I was pretty blue about the whole deal.

"A few days before the operation I met with a nurse who was trained to help people deal with colostomies. Again, at first, I kind of tuned her out too. But gradually she got through to me. It dawned on me what she was saying—that this can be managed. Yes, it takes some getting used to, and it takes work, and there will be times when it can be a first-class drag. But thousands of people have figured out how to cope with it. And there's no reason I couldn't either.

"Eventually, I got the message. Instead of letting this thing ruin my life, I decided I had thirty or forty more good years ahead of me, and I was going to live as normally as possible. It was the best decision I ever made.

"After the operation, the nurse worked with me to find the right kind of pouch and attachments for me. The pouch lies pretty flat, so I can wear the kinds of clothes I like. I can take the bag off and enjoy a hot shower, just like I always did. I had to tinker with my diet a little— I cut out eggs and cabbage, and some other things that seemed to increase gas. I still work out, but I don't use the weight machines any more. And since my cancer has been cured, I have less to worry about, so my attitude about a lot of things is healthier. I've even knocked a couple of strokes off my golf game.

"I've told some of my close friends about my ostomy, but other friends and most of the people I work with don't even know. I figure it's none of their business. But if anyone asks, I try to answer their questions as honestly as I can.

"And Rachel has been a real tower of strength. She helps me take care of the opening and the equipment sometimes, which is a real blessing if I've had a long day or am just not up to it. Once in a while she comes with me to my ostomy support group meetings. It's done us both good to be able to talk with other couples who are wrestling with these same problems.

"If anything, this experience helped us grow closer. Sex is just as good as it ever was. A while ago we started reading long books out loud to each other. We're in the middle of *David Copperfield* right now. That's our way of telling each other we're both in this thing for the long haul."

Chapter 9

Chemotherapy, Radiation, and Other Treatments

The strategy of using drugs or radiation (or both), in addition to surgery, for the treatment of colorectal cancer is known as adjuvant therapy. Adjuvant methods increase the chances that primary treatment will result in a cure. Drugs and radiation can reach and destroy cancer cells that may be left in the body after surgery has removed the main tumor. Adjuvant treatment can significantly delay the recurrence of cancer and may add years to life.

Within the past decade, adjuvant therapy has become the accepted method for helping just about everyone with Stage III colorectal cancer. (Remember that Stage III means the cancer has spread from the colon into the nearby lymph nodes.) In addition, most doctors now recommend adjuvant therapy for people with Stage II cancer who are at high risk of a recurrence at the original site (local recurrence).

Adjuvant therapy is sometimes given prior to surgery. This strategy (called neoadjuvant therapy) is intended to shrink the tumor and make it easier to remove. More often, additional treatment is administered after surgery to destroy any cancerous cells left behind during the operation. In some cases, adjuvant treatment can take place both before and after surgery.

CHEMOTHERAPY FOR ADVANCED
COLORECTAL CANCER

Chemotherapy means the use of chemicals (drugs) to treat disease. In a sense, any use of medicine is chemotherapy, but the word usually refers to cancer treatment. Substances used for this purpose are called anticancer drugs. Those that specifically kill cancer cells are known as cytotoxic drugs. Use of more than one drug at a time is called combination chemotherapy.

The main drug used in colorectal cancer is 5-fluorouracil, or 5-FU (also called Adrucil). 5-FU is also used for treatment of cancers in other parts of the body, including the breast, stomach, pancreas, bladder, prostate, and lung. Studies conducted on large numbers of patients at several major treatment centers show that treatment with 5-FU, in combination with surgery, significantly reduces the risk that colorectal cancer will recur. It also increases the length of survival.

To increase its effectiveness, 5-FU is usually given in combination with one of a group of additional drugs. These drugs do not work against cancer directly. Instead, they increase the cancer-killing power of the 5-FU.

Until very recently, the drug usually given in combination with 5-FU for adjuvant therapy was levamisole. This drug is used as a treatment for intestinal parasites and it appears to stimulate the immune system, but by itself it has no direct impact on cancer. Levamisole comes in pill form and is taken by mouth.

More recent studies provide convincing evidence that better results are achieved with a substance called leucovorin (also called calcium folinate). Leucovorin enhances the effectiveness of 5-FU by blocking enzymes that help cancer cells reproduce. Research has shown that people with Stage III colon cancer who take a combination of 5-FU and leucovorin after surgery have up to a 33 percent better chance of staying alive for five years or more, compared to those treated with surgery alone. The risk of recurrence also decreases by 41 percent with this combination. Since about 1996, this approach has become the standard adjuvant treatment in the United States.

Recent studies suggest that the combination of 5-FU and leucovorin, if given for six months, is as effective as 5-FU and levamisole given for a full year. A three-way combination (5-FU, leucovorin, and levamisole) may also significantly improve the survival rate, but this three-drug regimen causes a higher incidence of side effects such as diarrhea and mouth sores.

When used for adjuvant treatment, the combination of 5-FU and leucovorin is administered by intravenous (IV) injection. When drugs are used in combination with radiation therapy for Stage III cancer, they are given in continuous infusion through a small pump that is attached to the body and delivers precisely measured amounts throughout the day. Drug treatment for advanced (Stage IV) cancer can be given either as an injection or through continuous infusion.

Typically, adjuvant chemotherapy begins three to five weeks after surgery for colorectal cancer and continues for a period of time, usually six months. Often, cancer drugs are given in cycles. For example, 5-FU injections might be taken every day for five days, followed by a break until the next month, when the five-day process is repeated. Your physicians and nurses will design a treatment regimen to meet your specific needs.

Side effects can occur with any drug, and the medications used for colorectal cancer are no exception. Side effects are the result of the drug's impact on healthy cells, especially those that, like cancer, grow or reproduce quickly. Such cells are found in the hair roots, the cells of the mouth and intestines, and the blood-forming tissue of the bone marrow.

The most common adverse reactions to 5-FU are diarrhea and sores in the mouth or lips. Sometimes, the drug can cause pain or itching at the site of the injection. Other less common side effects include fever, chills, and stomach cramps. In rare cases, side effects include blood in the urine or stools, pinpoint red spots on the skin, and unusual bleeding or bruising. This drug often causes temporary loss of hair. Once the course of treatment is over, how-ever, hair usually grows back.

Leucovorin can also cause side effects, including mild nausea, vomiting, and diarrhea. When used in combination with 5-FU, it may cause damage to the bone marrow, which clears up after treatment ends. Skin rashes can also be a problem.

Most side effects disappear when treatment is stopped or mod-ified. If you experience any unexpected consequences of treat-ment, be sure to tell your care providers. You'll find the chemotherapy nurses especially helpful in this regard. There are remedies for many side effects; for example, some recently devel-oped drugs that can be given along with the chemotherapy will alleviate most, if not all, nausea and vomiting.

RADIATION THERAPY

Radiation therapy is the medical use of high-energy waves, some-what like X-rays, to treat disease. The rays penetrate inside the body and disrupt the activity of the cells. Radiation affects all the cells that lie within the treatment area. Normal, healthy cells will regrow quickly, but cancerous cells die or become unable to re-produce. Because radiation can damage normal cells, doctors try to use the lowest effective doses and to aim the waves as precisely as possible.

Radiation therapy (also called radiotherapy or irradiation) is an appropriate choice for people with cancers of the rectum. Use of radiotherapy can:

- Prevent local recurrence of the tumor;
- Arrest cancer that is spreading to other sites in the body;
- Reduce symptoms such as pressure, pain, or bleeding;
- Improve the long-term survival rate.

Radiation is generally used for treating cancer in the rectum. It is less often used as treatment for cancer in the colon. However, if a colon tumor appears to be too large to be surgically removable, radiation can shrink the tumor, allowing potentially curative surgery to take place.

The usual method of treating rectal cancer is external-beam radiation. The name refers to the fact that the rays come from a device positioned outside the body, somewhat like the X-ray machine a dentist uses. In rare cases of rectal cancer, doctors may decide to use a form of internal radiation, in which radioactive "seeds" are implanted in or near the tumor. Another approach, known as the Papillon technique, delivers a focused dose of radiation directly to the affected area. This method is effective but not widely available.

In some cases, radiation may be the only treatment given for rectal cancer. Usually, though, surgery is also performed. Radiation can be administered before or after the operation, or at both times, but after-surgery use is the most common strategy for treating rectal cancer in this country.

In a few treatment centers, high doses of radiation might be given during surgery. This approach, known as intraoperative radiation, is used when surgeons know in advance that they cannot remove a tumor completely. After the surgeon takes out as much of the cancer as possible, the therapist aims the radiation beam at the surgical site to destroy any cancerous cells left behind.

Drugs may also be given, along with radiation, either before or after surgery. This combined treatment is sometimes called chemoradiation.

In cases where extensive surgery would destroy the muscles of the anus (the sphincter), radiation plus limited surgery can bring the tumor under control while keeping the sphincter intact. This method may avoid the need for a permanent colostomy.

The total dose of radiation needed to treat rectal cancer is too high to be given all at once. Doing so would damage too much healthy tissue. Instead, the dose is divided into smaller units that are administered over the course of time, usually five days a week for five weeks. (Palliative therapy, given to relieve symptoms, may last only two or three weeks.) Therapy is not given on weekends so that the healthy cells can have a chance to recover. Dividing the dosage in this way is called fractionated radiation therapy.

Radiation is measured in units called "centigrays" (abbreviated cGy). The total dose used in treating rectal cancer is usually 4,500–5,000 cGy. To reach this total dose, fractionated doses of 180 to 200 cGy per day are given over a five-week period. In most treatment centers, the dose is administered once a day, but it is also possible to use smaller ("hyperfractionated") doses and give them several times a day at four- or six-hour intervals.

Radiation treatment is often handled by a team of medical professionals:

- The radiation oncologist (or radiation therapist), a physician who specializes in using this approach for the treatment of cancer, determines the type and amount of treatment needed and administers the dose.
- A radiation therapy nurse provides hands-on nursing care and education.
- A radiation physicist is in charge of running the equipment.
- A dosimetrist is responsible for calculating the number and timing of treatments.

Depending on your needs, the team may also include a dietitian, a physical therapist, a social worker, and others who can provide additional care and support.

Before you receive your first dose, your caregivers need to do some careful planning. You will be asked to undergo a simulation: you lie on a table while a special X-ray machine identifies the area of the body to be treated. The therapist will then mark the area with a special ink. (Be careful not to wash off these marks; they will be used to guide the radiation machines throughout the course of treatment.) The simulation test can take up to two hours.

A few days later, you will come in for your first dose. Special shields will be placed on your body to protect areas that should not be exposed to radiation. Sometimes, a kind of "body cast" is made to help you remain still. The treatment itself lasts only about a minute; the whole process may take about ten to fifteen minutes each time. Most people do not feel anything during the treatment; others notice a warm feeling. You will be alone in the treatment room, but your caregivers, who are operating the equipment in an adjoining room, can see and hear you at all times.

Treatment with radiation can cause side effects. Short-term (or acute) side effects include fatigue, changes in skin, and loss of appetite. Nausea and diarrhea may also occur, and some people experience increased frequency of urination due to irritation of the bladder. Usually, these problems get better in the weeks after therapy stops. Hair loss is not common following radiation treatment for rectal cancer. If the side effects are severe, your doctors may suggest taking a break from treatment for a week or so. Radiation treatment can lower your resistance to infection, so it is especially important to try and avoid catching colds or other illnesses during this period.

The effectiveness of radiation therapy can often be improved when 5-FU is administered at the same time. Recent studies suggest that this combination can lower the risk of local recurrence by 50 percent and can increase the length of disease-free survival compared to radiation therapy alone, whether radiation is given before or after surgery. Scientists are not yet sure why this combination works, but it appears that radiation alters cancer cells in such a way as to increase the cancer-killing ability of the 5-FU. For best results, the drug is continuously infused. A small portable pump attached to the body delivers small amounts of medication around the clock, usually for five weekdays, followed by a weekend "rest" period.

The combination of external-beam radiation and chemotherapy is also a good choice for treatment of anal cancers. In some cases, use of 5-FU plus the drugs mitomycin or cisplatin can cause some anal tumors to shrink so much that surgery may be unnecessary. Occasionally, local excision (removal of residual tumor) may be all that is required. This approach avoids more extensive surgery, which may involve removing the tumor and the surrounding tissues, blood vessels, and lymph vessels and usually requires a permanent colostomy. Some evidence suggests that using drugs and then administering radiation may be more effective in treating anal cancer than giving both treatments simultaneously. Your doctors will choose the approach that offers the best results in your circumstances.

Researchers are also exploring the use of additional drugs that can boost the effectiveness of radiation even further. These medications are known as radiosensitizers.

STAGE IV DISEASE

The adjuvant strategies discussed above produce good results in people with Stage III colorectal cancer. Treatment of metastatic (Stage IV) colorectal cancer using these methods is usually less effective. Between 10 and 20 percent of people who take 5-FU plus leucovorin might experience some short-term relief of symptoms. Some individuals may experience palliation through use of radiation therapy.

The combination of 5-FU and leucovorin represents what doctors call "first-line" adjuvant drug therapy for colorectal cancer. In 1996, the U.S. Food and Drug Administration (FDA) approved a new injectable drug called irinotecan (sold under the name Camptostar and manufactured by Pharmacia & Upjohn). This compound, promoted as the only new drug for colorectal cancer in forty years, is best considered as a "second-line" treatment. Irinotecan is not a cure. Its use is reserved for patients who do not show any response to standard therapy for advanced disease or who did respond but whose cancer is now progressing again. Studies show that about 15 percent of people who use irinotecan experience a reduction in tumor size of 50 percent or more. However, this response may last only a short time—around four months or so. Possible side effects include severe diarrhea, loss of white blood cells, hair loss, and increased risk of infection, nausea, and vomiting. The drug should not be taken at the same time as other anticancer drugs, such as cis-platin, because the combination can be fatal.

EXPERIMENTAL TREATMENTS

Monoclonal Antibodies

Antibodies are proteins produced by cells of the immune system. These proteins recognize and respond to the presence of dangerous substances in the body, including infectious particles or abnormal cells such as cancerous cells. Each antibody is designed to recognize one and only one type of invader.

In the laboratory, scientists can manufacture specific kinds of these proteins, known as monoclonal antibodies. It is possible to attach certain molecules, such as drugs or radioactive particles, to these antibodies and inject the compound into the body. The antibodies then circulate until they find their target and bind to it. Once attached in this way, they release their "cargo," delivering the drug directly to the site. In a way, this strategy is like creating "smart bombs" that can be programmed to seek out and destroy specific targets, such as cancerous cells.

Research is being conducted to determine whether monoclonal antibodies can be designed that will deliver anticancer drugs directly to the cells of a colorectal cancer tumor. Studies on a monoclonal antibody called 17-1A as adjuvant treatment suggest that this treatment may reduce the rates of recurrence and mortality of Stage III colorectal cancer by around 30 percent, compared to surgery alone. The benefits appear to be about the same as with conventional chemotherapy drugs, but there is a lower incidence of toxic side effects. Widespread use of this therapy lies in the future, but early research indicates that it has promise. Clinical trials are in progress in the United States and Europe.

Immunotherapy

The body's immune system protects against infections and other illnesses. In many instances, the cells of the immune system can launch an attack against cancerous cells and prevent tumors from developing and spreading. Research is under way to find methods of enhancing the natural immune activity so that it can help fend off the progression and spread of cancer. This approach is called immunotherapy. At this time, results of immunotherapy in treating colorectal cancer have been disappointing.

Gene Therapy

As you learned in Chapter 3, genes are the basic units of heredity. A gene is a fragment of DNA that controls the activity in the body's cells, including cancer cells. If a gene becomes damaged, it can trigger the onset of cancer. Damaged genes are sometimes passed on to the next generation, increasing the risk that the offspring will inherit a tendency to develop certain kinds of colorectal cancer.

Gene therapy refers to the use of genes in the treatment of diseases such as cancer. In some cases, researchers can repair a damaged or missing gene in a cell by replacing it with a "healthy" or complete chunk of normal DNA. Another approach is to create drugs that can be administered. Once inside the body, these drugs serve the same function as the missing or defective gene.

The science of gene therapy is still very new. Additional studies may determine whether it will be of value in treating cancers of the colon, rectum, and anus.

CLINICAL TRIALS

To learn whether a type of treatment is effective, scientists conduct studies following strict rules of research. They then subject the results from those studies to careful analysis. The main questions they want to answer are:

- Does this treatment work?
- Does it work better than other treatments already available?
- What side effects does the treatment cause?
- Do the benefits outweigh the risks, including side effects?
- In which patients is the treatment most likely to be helpful?

Studies involving promising new or experimental therapies in human patients are known as *clinical trials*. These trials are carried out in phases, with each phase designed to find out certain information. Which phase you participate in depends on your general condition and the type and stage of your cancer.

A number of drugs are currently being evaluated in clinical trials. Carboxamine-amino-imidazole (CAI) is a drug that interferes with the ability of cancer cells to metastasize. In the laboratory, CAI blocks the growth of several types of cancers, including colon cancer. Whether it works in humans, without causing an unacceptably high rate of side effects, is now under investigation.

THE PHASES OF CLINICAL TRIALS

In a Phase I study, the goal is to see whether the treatment can be given safely to humans and in what doses. The substance has already been tested in laboratory animals. Researchers administer the treatment according to strict guidelines (protocols) and watch carefully for any harmful side effects. Because the safety of the treatment for humans is not known, Phase I studies may involve significant risks. The patients who take part in these studies are usually those whose cancer has spread and who are not likely to be helped by other known treatments.

Once the Phase I study determines the safety and dosage of the treatment, Phase II studies are conducted to determine whether the treatment has any real effect on the cancer. Depending on the study design, scientists measure such outcomes as tumor shrinkage, rate of metastasis, reduction in symptoms, or overall improvements in quality of life.

If a treatment has shown activity against cancer in Phase II, it moves to Phase III. Here, the new therapy is compared with the standard treatment to see which is more effective. Because of the slow-growing nature of colorectal cancer, and the fact that benefit is measured in increased survival times, such studies often require years of effort before the results are known.

In Phase III studies for new treatments for colorectal cancer, patients are divided into two groups. One receives the new treatment and the other receives standard adjuvant therapy (that is, 5-FU and leucovorin, or radiation, or both). Because we now have solid proof that use of adjuvant treatment for Stage III colorectal cancer is beneficial, patients in clinical trials are not given placebos (harmless but ineffective treatments). The results of the two treatments are compared, and the researchers publish their findings in scientific journals. Often, another team of investigators will conduct a similar experiment to see whether they achieve the same results. Eventually, doctors reach some consensus on whether the treatment is worth giving to their patients.

Phase IV studies (sometimes called postmarketing studies) take place after the new treatment has been made available for sale to all doctors and treatment centers, not just those taking part in the research. These studies involve data on hundreds, even thousands, of patients using the treatment in the "real world" of clinical practice. Depending on the results, a treatment in Phase IV studies may become part of standard treatment in patient care.

During your course of treatment, your physician may suggest that you take part in a clinical trial of one of these investigational drugs. This does not mean you are being asked to serve merely as a human "guinea pig." A clinical trial is only undertaken when there is some evidence suggesting that the treatment being studied may indeed be of value.

Nor does being offered a clinical trial mean your case is hopeless and your physicians are suggesting a last-ditch effort. Drugs used in clinical trials are often found to provide real benefits.

However, there are some risks. No one involved in the study knows in advance whether the treatment will work or what side effects will occur. That's what the study is designed to discover. Most side effects will disappear in time, but some can be permanent or even life-threatening. Remember, too, that even standard treatments have side effects. Depending on many factors, you may decide that a clinical trial will be of value in your case.

People who take part in these studies do so for a number of reasons. Naturally, they hope that the treatment will help them. They may hope for a cure of the disease, a longer time to live, a way to feel better. But they also may participate because they know they are making an important contribution to medical care.

Enrollment in any clinical trial is completely voluntary. Your doctors and nurses will explain the study to you in detail and will give you a form to read. If you sign it, you are indicating your desire to take part. This process is known as obtaining informed consent. Even if you sign the form and the trial begins, you are free to leave the study any time you want, for any reason. Taking part in the study does not prevent you from getting other medical care you may need.

To find out more about clinical trials, talk to your physicians. Among the questions you should ask are:

- What is the purpose of the study?
- What kinds of tests and treatments does the study involve?
- What does this treatment do?
- What is likely to happen in my case, with or without this new research treatment?
- What are my other choices and what are their advantages and disadvantages?
- How could the study affect my daily life?
- What side effects can I expect from the study?
- How long will the study last?
- Will I have to be hospitalized? If so, how often and for how long?

- Will the study cost me anything? Will any of the treatment be free?
- If I am harmed as a result of the research, what treatment would I be entitled to?
- What type of long-term follow-up care is part of the study?

The "Resources" section at the back of this book contains suggestions on how to find out more about these programs.

A WORD ABOUT PAIN

Understandably, for many people, the greatest fear associated with cancer is that they will suffer pain, either because of the disease or because of the treatment. Pain is a serious complication. It can rob people of their energy and their enjoyment of life. It also interferes with their ability to undergo or comply with treatment, which increases the risk that the cancer may get worse. To be complete, treatment for colorectal cancer needs to address the problem of pain.

Cancer pain can result from the effects of a tumor that penetrates through tissue and invades or presses on nearby nerves. In colorectal cancer, tumors that block the intestine can cause pain. Pain associated with cancer is of two main types, acute and chronic. Acute (sudden or short-lived) pain can result from tissue damage. Usually, this kind of pain can be easily treated and it goes away after a while. Chronic pain may result from the progression of the disease or from treatment. Over time, the nerves become desensitized to the pain. In such cases, the "hurt" caused by pain may diminish, but the pain may show up in the form of depression, anxiety, or sleeplessness.

Fortunately, there is effective treatment for pain associated with cancer. If you experience pain at any time during the course of your illness or its therapy, don't be afraid to speak up. Let your caregivers know. In recent years, cancer specialists have become increasingly aware of the importance of managing pain as a way to improve the quality of their patients' lives. But they can't know that you are suffering unless you tell them.

Treatment for cancer pain is administered in three steps:

- Step 1, aimed at mild cancer pain, depends on medications that do not contain narcotics. Options include analgesic drugs, including nonsteroidal anti-inflammatory drugs (NSAIDs) such as aspirin or ibuprofen, or other pain relievers such as acetaminophen (Tylenol*). In some cases, medications such as antidepressants or antihistamines may also help.
- Step 2 involves pain that persists or increases. At this point, a combination of pain relievers, including a weak opioid drug such as codeine, may be tried, along with other types of medications.
- Step 3 relies on strong opioids such as morphine, often in combination with NSAIDs and other drugs that can relieve symptoms, such as the steroid dexamethasone.

Besides pill form, drugs for severe pain can be given in several ways. Small electronic pumps worn on the body are controlled by the patient to deliver small regular doses whenever needed. Also available is a skin patch (similar to the patch used to curb cigarette smoking) that contains doses of a pain reliever called fentanyl, which is absorbed slowly through the skin to provide around-the-clock pain relief.

Some people resist taking narcotic medications because they are afraid of becoming addicted. Studies show this is not likely to happen, even when the patient uses a pump or other means to control the dose of medication. The benefits of pain therapy far outweigh this concern. With prolonged usage, patients may develop a tolerance to a drug, which means that larger doses may be

*Tylenol: McNeil

needed to provide the same level relief. Tolerance is not the same as addiction or dependence. If you are concerned about this issue, discuss it with your caregivers.

In addition to drugs, there are other options for pain management, depending on the source and nature of the problem. For many people, surgery, radiation, or procedures to deaden nerve sensitivity may work. Behavioral techniques such as art or music therapy, relaxation exercises, biofeedback, and imagery can also help reduce the stress and tension associated with cancer and its treatment. Cancer pain is a real problem; it is not "all in your head." Even so, many people find that talking to a psychological counselor or a psychiatrist helps them cope with their situation.

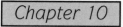

Chapter 10

Alternative and Complementary Therapies

Conventional therapy is the term doctors use in referring to established treatments for cancer. Their value has been demonstrated in rigorous scientific studies, and they are available from licensed medical professionals. The treatments described in the preceding chapters are conventional therapies.

As you continue to learn more about your colorectal cancer, friends or family members, articles in magazines, or reports on television or radio may suggest other types of therapies that are available outside the mainstream of medicine. These approaches may involve anything from simple dietary supplements to complex and costly therapies requiring stays of several months at clinics in foreign countries.

Such therapies go by various names. The most common term, *alternative therapy*, indicates that the treatment is different from standard medical approaches. *Unproven therapy* means that the treatment's usefulness has not yet been established through rigorous scientific study. Another label sometimes used is *questionable treatment*. To a certain extent, these terms can be used interchangeably. For example, most alternative therapies also happen to be unproven. In this chapter, for the sake of simplicity, I will refer to all such approaches as *alternative therapies*.

Complementary therapy—a treatment that might add to or support any benefits derived from conventional medicine— is different from alternative therapy. Generally, the term refers to psychological or supportive therapies, such as biofeedback, counseling, group sessions, meditation, massage, and so on. Complementary approaches usually do not involve the use of drugs or invasive techniques. They are not aimed at treating cancer per se but they seek to improve one's overall state of well-being and comfort. A therapy can be an alternative and a complementary one depending on how it is used. For example, aroma therapy, as a fragrance added to a warm bath or massage, can be soothing and relaxing. But if used as an alternative, aroma therapy will not cure colorectal cancer.

If you are curious about alternative or complementary treatments or any other strategies, by all means talk to your cancer care providers. You have the right to receive complete, accurate, and up-to-date information about any subject that is on your mind. Don't feel hesitant or embarrassed. In conversations with your doctors and other professionals, you can learn about the available options and find out whether any of them might offer benefits in your circumstances. If your caregivers are unable or unwilling to discuss the subject with you, ask them to put you in touch with someone who will.

Within the past few years, the United States government has taken important steps to encourage more research into alternative therapies. A new department within the National Institutes of Health, the Office of Alternative Medicine (OAM), distributes grants to scientists who design research projects to evaluate non-traditional methods of healing. The ultimate goal is to integrate into the standard medical approaches any alternative therapies that are found to be of value. Some types of alternative treatments are listed in the box on page 160. Information about one of the OAM-funded sites, the University of Texas Center for Alternative Medicine Research in Cancer, appears in the "Resources" section at the back of this book.

TYPES OF ALTERNATIVE THERAPIES

Category	Examples
Folk/ethnic therapies	Asian medicine ayurvedic medicine herbal medicine homeopathic medicine Native American medicine
Nutritional therapies	diet supplements macrobiotics megavitamins fasting and juice therapies
Mind/body control therapies	biofeedback guided imagery hypnotherapy music/sound therapy prayer therapy relaxation
Pharmacological and biological therapies	antioxidants cell treatment chelation therapy metabolic therapy oxidizing agents
Structural manipulations/ Energetic therapies	acupunctive acupressure chiropractic medicine electromagnetic therapies massage Qi Gong reflexology Rolfing therapeutic touch

MACROBIOTIC DIET

A macrobiotic diet is based on an ancient Asian philosophy that strives to achieve balance between the opposing forces that exist in the universe (known as yin and yang). According to this way of thinking, foods such as sugar, citrus fruits, spices, and so on, are classified as yin, and animal foods are classified as yang. As defined by the "founder" of the macrobiotic diet, George Ohsawa, a standard macrobiotic diet consists of 50 to 60 percent rice and whole-grain cereals, 20 to 25 percent vegetables, 5 to 10 percent beans and sea vegetables, and 5 percent soups. Liquids are to be consumed sparingly.

Some people believe that certain cancers can be defined as yin or yang, depending on foods that supposedly caused the tumors. For example, breast cancer is classified as more of a yin cancer, and colon cancer is more yang. The macrobiotic diet attempts to restore balance by emphasizing consumption of the "opposite" foods. For example, a diet for colon cancer calls for avoiding buckwheat and using milder flavoring and seasoning, more light cooking, and more leafy green vegetables.

In recent years, many people have claimed that a macrobiotic diet works to prevent cancer and to treat existing cancer. As is the case with many alternative therapies, however, scientific evidence to evaluate this claim does not exist. There is also concern that such a diet may be nutritionally unsound. For example, the diet does not usually provide the calories an adult needs each day for energy. One study, for example, found that adults following a macrobiotic diet had an average intake of only 60 to 70 percent of the recommended daily intake of calories. A macrobiotic diet typically does not provide enough of certain nutrients, such as protein, to provide balanced nutrition. Many people who eat such a diet lose weight—a key concern for people with cancer, because weight loss can mean a poorer prognosis.

Although the macrobiotic diet is nutritionally unsound, vegetarian diets can be made nutritionally adequate with sufficient planning. Lower consumption of animal fats and higher consumption of vegetables and fruits can lower the risk of colorectal cancer. Such a diet, however, does not have any effect on established, metastatic colorectal cancer.

The smartest approach is to find out all you can about *any* treatment, standard or alternative, before you decide to accept it. Also, be sure to let your medical team know if you are undergoing any form of alternative therapy now or plan to start in the future. Do not change or drop out of traditional medical treatment without speaking to your caregivers first. You have the right to make such decisions, but you will need advice and guidance on how to make any changes in the safest way possible.

THE APPEAL OF ALTERNATIVE THERAPIES

Surveys show that one cancer patient in ten tries an alternative treatment at some point in the course of care. The appeal that alternative therapies have for people coping with colorectal cancer—or cancer of any kind, for that matter—is understandable. Cancer is a serious, frightening, and life-threatening disease. People want to do everything they can to get better, to avoid pain and suffering, and to prolong their lives. If the disease is not diagnosed until it has reached an advanced stage, or if gets worse despite treatment, the urge to try something other than conventional therapy is very great.

People also explore alternative approaches because traditional treatment for colorectal cancer clearly has its share of drawbacks. Surgery poses risks. Radiation is inconvenient. Chemotherapy can cause serious side effects. All these therapies are expensive. Naturally, we hope that any potential benefits of these treatments—complete cure, longer life—outweigh any risks. But there are no guarantees. Conventional treatments don't always work. Despite the best efforts of a team of dedicated professionals using the most up-to-date methods available, most people with advanced colorectal cancer will die of their disease.

Some people try alternative approaches because they feel their doctors have decided their case is hopeless and there is nothing left to do. There may indeed come a point where all the traditional treatment options have been tried. Even so, hope remains that a clinical trial of a new therapy may yield good results. And treatment is always available to address pain or other complications of advanced disease.

Nowadays, many people want to take a more active role in their medical treatment. Alternative therapies offer them a chance to do so.

People who are dissatisfied with their treatment may blame "the medical establishment"—doctors, governments, and pharmaceutical companies—for deliberately withholding information about the latest miracle cure. It is impossible for every physician to stay absolutely up-to-date with the current research on every treatment. But no ethical doctor would deny patients access to any legal therapy when there is solid evidence that its use may provide at least *some* benefit, especially after conventional treatments have been exhausted.

Admittedly, doctors' attitudes sometimes contribute to the problem. As specialists, we may become very intent on removing a tumor or destroying the last cancerous cell lurking in a patient's body. In focusing on the disease, we may neglect to consider the whole person—thoughts, feelings, emotions, the overall impact of the disease and its treatment on a person's life, and the lives of friends, family, and neighbors. Until recently, traditional medicine has not always emphasized the importance of good nutrition, exercise, and mental attitudes as important aspects of medical care. Promoters of holistic therapies—treatments aimed at the whole person, in body, mind, and spirit—have stepped in to fill the void.

THE DRAWBACKS AND LIMITATIONS OF ALTERNATIVE AND COMPLEMENTARY TREATMENTS

The biggest concern is that an alternative therapy may make a disease worse, either directly (by causing the disease to progress or spread) or indirectly (by interfering with or preventing treatment that might have done some good). The time and money spent on untested, unsafe, or worthless alternatives is better invested in a conventional therapy that has been demonstrated to offer help to at least some people. And some alternative medications can have uncomfortable, painful, or even life-threatening side effects.

For patients trying to cope with a serious illness, dealing concurrently with alternative care and traditional care can be confusing. Because effective conventional therapies can cause side effects, some people mistakenly believe everything "bad" that happens to them is due to their medical treatment, and everything "good" is the result of an alternative approach.

Without doubt, good nutrition—adequate intake of calories, proteins, and other nutrients—is important for everyone. Exercise keeps the body strong and functioning at peak efficiency. Positive attitudes are invaluable assets in the fight against cancer. Spiritual pursuits infuse life with joy and meaning. *But these things, by themselves, simply will not stop colorectal cancer from progressing.* Effective medical treatment that will stop tumors from growing and spreading is also needed. This is why the combination of effective conventional anticancer treatment with complementary therapies involving a balanced diet, various forms of exercise, relaxation techniques or spirituality makes perfect sense to many patients. In some situations, these complementary therapies can have a very positive impact on relieving symptoms and improving quality of life.

EVALUATING THE CLAIMS

Conventional treatments only become standard after they have been subjected to years of research. Before a drug, device, or procedure becomes available on the market, it undergoes rigorous evaluation. Data from these studies are published in journals and presented at scientific meetings, so they can be discussed and debated. Other researchers often try to repeat an experiment to see whether they get the same results. This long and complex process allows other qualified experts to evaluate the researchers' claims. Then the U.S. Food and Drug Administration (FDA) conducts a careful review of all the available data. If the FDA is not satisfied that studies support the claims of safety and efficacy, it will either order further tests to be conducted or it will refuse to allow the product to be marketed. Only if the treatment passes this intense scrutiny will the FDA approve it for use in patients. Even after

QUESTIONS FOR EVALUATING A THERAPY

- Has the treatment been evaluated in clinical trials? A reference librarian can help you find out whether a particular treatment has been reported in reputable scientific journals.
- Do the practitioners of an approach claim that the medical community is trying to keep their cure from the public? No one genuinely committed to finding better ways to treat a disease would knowingly keep an effective treatment a secret or try to suppress such a treatment.
- Does the treatment rely on nutritional or diet therapy as its main focus? At this time, there is no known dietary cure for cancer. In other words, there is no evidence that diet alone can get rid of cancerous cells in the body.
- Do those who endorse the treatment claim that it is harmless and painless and that it produces no unpleasant side effects? Because treatments for cancer must be very powerful, they frequently have unpleasant side effects.
- Does the treatment have a "secret formula" that only a small group of practitioners can use? Scientists who believe they have developed an effective treatment routinely publish their results in reputable peer-reviewed journals so they can be evaluated by other researchers.

Source: The National Cancer Institute

the therapy is available, research continues, to make sure the benefits continue to outweigh the risks.

The claims made for the safety and effectiveness of alternative treatments are not tested by this same process. Many who advocate these treatments simply state that their drug or their method works, that it produces a complete cure even in cases traditional doctors have called hopeless, and that it has no side effects. Often, these promoters refuse to disclose the contents of their medication. The reason they give is: they are afraid that others will steal their secret formula. In reality, their formula may contain worthless or harmful substances that offer no real benefit and may interfere with conventional therapy.

If you or a loved one is curious about an alternative form of treatment, read the questions in the accompanying box before trying it.

Chapter 11

Eating Right

As you learned in Chapter 4, colon and rectal cancers are among the most preventable forms of the disease. Because certain foods can raise the risk of cancer, it makes sense that adjusting the diet can lower the risk.

But, for most of us, making changes in our eating habits can be very hard. After all, we're only human, and we naturally prefer to eat foods that we like. It's no surprise that high-fat foods—ice cream, meats, crispy snacks—often taste very good. Food choices also become habits. We buy products we already know, we order similar things in restaurants. We are also creatures of daily routines. It takes less time and causes less stress to do things the way we've always done them. With our busy schedules, it's easier to prepare familiar or traditional meals than it is to spend hours shopping and experimenting with complicated recipes. Parents find it a huge challenge to serve meals that will appeal to picky eaters and still meet the nutritional needs of children and adults who are trying to watch what they eat. Our culture is another factor. Store shelves are crammed with "convenience" foods. Americans eat many of their meals away from home. Fast-food restaurants, with many high-fat items on the menu, pop up on every corner. It can be hard to follow a careful diet when traveling or when visiting friends and relatives. Lavish (and not always wholesome) meals are a key part of many events, from holidays and celebrations to business meetings and backyard barbecues.

Despite these many obstacles, it is still possible to eat right. As scientific evidence mounts that a proper diet significantly lowers the risk of cancer and other major diseases, more people are demanding easier access to healthier foods. Many grocery stores now make it easier to buy fresher, high-fiber foods and lower-fat products, including favorite snack foods and prepackaged meals. Restaurant menus feature special low-fat and "heart-healthy" entrees. Airlines offer a variety of meals to customers who request them. And countless healthy recipes are available, not just in cookbooks but also through the Internet. (See "For Further Reading," pages 236–238.) This chapter contains a sample of recipes to help you get started.

If you're like most people, your chances of success are greater if you change your eating habits gradually, rather than make huge changes all at once. The three main goals are: (1) increase the amount of fiber from vegetables, fruits, and beans, (2) use whole grains when possible, and (3) lower fat intake.

INCREASE INTAKE OF FRUITS AND VEGETABLES

Nutritionists recommend eating at least five servings of fruits and vegetables every day. A serving can be a 6-ounce glass of juice, ½ cup of cut-up fruits or vegetables, 1 medium piece of fruit, 1 cup of leafy vegetables, ½ cup of cooked dried peas or beans, and/or ¼ cup of dried fruit. Here are some tips for reaching the five-a-day target:

- Buy a large selection of fruits and vegetables when you shop. You will have lots of variety and some will always be on hand when you need them. Fresh is best, but canned and frozen products can be valuable too. Canned beans and peas are convenient and easy to use.
- Use the fresh fruits and vegetables that spoil quickest (berries, bananas, peaches, and asparagus) as soon as possible after purchase. Use hardier varieties (apples, squash, and so on) and frozen or canned products later in the week.

- Many stores sell cut-up vegetables and fruits in a "salad-bar" display. This a convenient way to select a variety of healthy foods. It is also a good option for lunches.
- Keep a fruit bowl and small packs of applesauce, raisins, or other dried fruit on your kitchen counter, dining table, or desk.
- Pack pieces of fruit or cut-up vegetables (carrots, peppers, and so on) in your briefcase or backpack.
- Keep a bowl of cut-up vegetables on a visible and easy-to-reach shelf in your refrigerator. Storing celery or carrot sticks in a jar with some water keeps them fresh, crisp, and cold.
- Start your intake of fruit at breakfast by drinking a glass of 100 percent juice, eating an orange or half a melon, or topping off your cereal with fruit (berries, raisins, peaches).
- Include a salad with your lunch or dinner. You can buy a variety of precut packaged salads that contain high-quality, fresh ingredients.
- Serve stir-fry or steamed vegetables (alone or with chicken pieces) as a main course.
- Have fruit as your dessert. Low-fat yogurt or sherbet topped with berries or melon is a good choice.
- Add extra vegetables to soups, sauces, and casseroles.
- Substitute beans for meat in such dishes as tacos, burritos, and chili.
- Serve soups containing beans or peas—minestrone, split-pea, black bean, or lentil soup—as main courses.
- Try black-eyed peas or black beans as side dishes.
- Add kidney beans or garbanzo beans (chickpeas) to fresh salads.

INCREASE INTAKE OF WHOLE GRAINS

As you learned in Chapter 4, whole grains contain much more fiber than processed or "refined" grain products because they retain the hull and the kernel (germ). To increase your consumption of these products:

- Choose bread and bakery products that have whole wheat, cracked wheat, or other whole grains as the first ingredient on the ingredient list.
- Buy whole-grain cereals.
- Select cereals that provide at least four grams of fiber per serving.
- In the winter months, enjoy whole-grain hot cereals such as oatmeal.
- Use whole wheat flour in cooking and baking. Choose the whole-grain variety of pancake and waffle mixes or frozen products.
- Replace at least half of the white flour with whole wheat flour in recipes.
- Serve whole wheat noodles, brown rice, or cracked wheat (bulgur) as side dishes for dinner.
- Try main dishes such as spinach lasagna made with whole-grain noodles, and red or black beans over brown rice.
- Select high-fiber snacks and crackers, such as whole-grain crackers and flatbreads.

REDUCE FAT

A reasonable goal is to consume no more than 30 percent of your calories in the form of fats and oils (approximately 65 grams of fat for a 2,000-calorie diet). To reach this target, consider adopting the following strategies:

- Use reduced-fat or nonfat salad dressings, or try lemon juice, dried herbs, sliced green onions, or salsa as a topping for salads and vegetables.
- Use nonfat spreads such as jelly or jam, fruit spread, apple butter, or mustard.

- Top baked potatoes with plain nonfat or low-fat yogurt, sour cream, cottage cheese, ranch-type salad dressing, salsa, or even vinegar.
- Cut back on servings of high-fat dressings such as butter, mayonnaise, sour cream, or salad toppings. Use reduced fat mayonnaise or margarine.
- Switch to 1 percent or fat-free milk.
- Use less cheese in sandwiches and cooking. Use lower-fat or fat-free cheeses (such as part-skim mozzarella) whenever possible.
- Resist high-calorie desserts or fried foods such as french fries except as occasional treats. Consider splitting an order of these items with your meal partner.
- Cut down on serving portions; trim fat from meat; remove skin from poultry.
- Select lower-fat luncheon meats such as sliced turkey or chicken breast, rather than pastrami or corned beef.

EATING RIGHT DURING AND AFTER TREATMENT

If you recently received treatment for colorectal cancer, or are in treatment now, eating right is especially important for you. Surgery, radiation, and chemotherapy, plus the emotional stress and physical strain of coping with this disease, all affect the body in different ways. You need to eat well so that you can maintain your strength, get the most out of your therapy, and prevent your cancer from recurring. Your cancer care team should include a registered dietitian who can advise you about proper eating during this crucial period of your life.

People who eat well during their treatment are better able to cope with the side effects of treatment. A healthy diet helps you keep up your strength, prevents body tissues from breaking down, and rebuilds tissues affected by cancer treatment. Good nutrition also keeps your immune system working properly to help you fight off infection. Generally, eating a balanced diet with adequate portions is all the "nutritional therapy" you need. Avoid taking nutritional supplements or starting on special or unusual diets, unless these have been specifically recommended by your care team.

Each type of treatment can affect your eating in different ways. Not surprisingly, having part of your intestine removed will cause changes in your digestion and in your bowel habits. The human body adapts very well, however. It is possible that after a few months your digestion will return to nearly normal. Chemotherapy and radiation can cause such side effects as nausea and vomiting, loss of appetite, diarrhea or constipation, sore mouth or throat, and changes in the way food tastes. Your nutrition counselors can suggest ways to adjust your eating habits to help you cope with these problems if they occur. For example, eating soft foods or special tasty and nutritious milk shakes can overcome soreness in the mouth or throat. Cooking with herbs and spices, or varying your menu, can perk up your taste buds and make food seem more appealing. The National Cancer Institute's booklet, "Eating Hints," offers many helpful suggestions about how to eat well during your cancer treatment.

MENUS

The strategies described in the above section are general guidelines for improving your diet. Following are some suggested menus that will incorporate those strategies into your daily meals. An asterisk (*) indicates that the recipe for this item appears in the next section of the chapter.

Breakfast

½ grapefruit
*Swiss Fruit Muesli
1 cup skim milk

Fiber—6.5 g
Fat—2 g
Calories—370

1 orange
*Breakfast Bar-and-Fruit Mix
1 slice whole wheat toast with
    1 teaspoon jam or jelly
1 cup skim milk

Fiber—11 g
Fat—8 g
Calories—510

6 ounces orange juice
Bran flakes with strawberries
*1 Refrigerator Bran Muffin (medium)
    with 1 teaspoon jam or jelly
1 cup skim milk

Fiber—9 g
Fat—7 g
Calories—430

3 stewed prunes
Shredded Wheat biscuit
1 boiled egg
1 slice whole wheat toast with
    ½ teaspoon butter or margarine
1 cup skim milk

Fiber—14 g
Fat—9 g
Calories—500

Lunch

Oven toasted cheese sandwich (1½ ounces
    reduced-fat milk cheese; 2 slices whole
    wheat bread)
½ cup carrot sticks
½ cup peaches packed in water
*Cinnamon Coffee Cake

Fiber—7.5 g
Fat—8 g
Calories—460

*Tricolor Bean Soup
*Whole Wheat Irish Soda Bread with   ⎧ Fiber—15 g
    1 teaspoon butter   ⎨ Fat—17 g
    ½ cup low-fat yogurt   ⎩ Calories—540
*2 Almond-Apricot Squares

*½ cup Bermuda Bean Salad
*1 Whole Wheat Raisin Scone   ⎧ Fiber—17 g
*Prune cake   ⎨ Fat—13 g
    1 cup skim milk   ⎩ Calories—800
    1 banana

Chicken sandwich on whole wheat bread with
    lettuce or alfalfa sprouts
    ½ cup celery sticks   ⎧ Fiber—9 g
    1 tangerine   ⎨ Fat—12 g
*Wheat Germ Crisp Cookies   ⎩ Calories—550
    1 cup skim milk

DINNER

*Chicken Dijon
    ¾ cup brown rice
    1 cup steamed asparagus   ⎧ Fiber—7 g
    Whole wheat roll with 1 teaspoon butter ⎨ Fat—15 g
*Rhubarb Crumb Pie   ⎩ Calories—800
    1 cup skim milk

*Marinated Flank Steak
*Mashed Potatoes with Onions   ⎧ Fiber—7 g
*Broccoli and Sweet Pepper Stir-Fry   ⎨ Fat—21 g
*Poached Pears with Chocolate Sauce   ⎩ Calories—610
    1 cup skim milk

*Sole Filets with Lemon and Parsley
Brown rice
Steamed green beans   Fiber—11 g
*Spinach Supper Salad   Fat—29 g
*Buttermilk Herb Dressing   Calories—640
Chocolate Cake
1 cup skim milk

*Old-Fashioned Meat Loaf
1 medium baked potato   Fiber—11 g
½ cup steamed brussels sprouts Fat—18 g
*½ cup Tarragon Carrots   Calories—660
*Clafouti (French Baked-Fruit Custard)
1 cup skim milk

*Baked Salmon with Herbs
½ cup fresh green peas with pepper and
    whipped butter
Whole wheat roll   Fiber—9 g
Garden salad (greens, carrots, broccoli, Fat—28 g
    kidney beans)   Calories—700
*Oil and Vinegar Dressing
1½ cups sliced strawberries

*Creamy Pasta with Broccoli, Cauliflower,
    and Mushrooms
Italian bread   Fiber—9 g
Garden salad (greens, carrots, broccoli, Fat—11 g
    kidney beans)   Calories—600
½ cantaloupe

*Fettuccine with Fresh Tomatoes and Basil
Garden salad (greens, carrots, broccoli, Fiber—11.5 g
    kidney beans)   Fat—22 g
Steamed vegetables   Calories—693
Garlic bread
Chocolate frozen yogurt

*Winter Vegetable Stew
  Corn bread
  Garden salad (greens, carrots, broccoli,
    kidney beans)
  Baked apple

Fiber—13 g
Fat—11 g
Calories—450

SNACKS

Item	Fiber (g)	Fat (g)	Calories
Apple (whole, with skin)	2.8	0.5	81
Applesauce (½ cup)	2.0	0.1	53
Banana	2.2	0.6	105
Carrot (1 raw)	2.3	0.1	31
Celery (1 stalk)	0.6	0.1	6
Cottage cheese (1% fat, ¼ cup)	0.0	0.6	41
Dried apricots (7)	2.1	0.0	63
Fig bar (2)	1.4	1.8	112
Fudgesicle	1.0	0.2	98
Grapes (1½ cups)	2.0	0.0	85
Melon (1 cup)	2.3	0.5	100
Orange (1)	3.1	0.2	62
Pear (1 whole)	4.3	0.7	98
Popcorn (3 cups, air popped)	3.6	1.2	93
Sherbet (½ cup)	0.0	2.0	136
Tuna (in water, 1 can)	0.0	1.1	47
Vanilla wafers (6)	0.2	4.8	102
Wheat bagel	4.3	0.7	153
Yogurt (nonfat with fruit, 1 cup)	1.1	0.5	100

RECIPES

Many people enjoy cooking; others find it a time-consuming chore. There's no rule that says you have to become a rival to Julia Child and create all of your meals from scratch. Shortcuts such as precut bagged salads, ready-made pie crusts, or soup starter kits are perfectly acceptable. The goal is to eat well, not to spend the rest of your life chained to your kitchen appliances.

These recipes originally appeared in *The American Cancer Society Cookbook,* by Anne Lindsay (New York: Hearst Books, 1988). They cover everything from soup to dessert, are pretty simple to prepare, and should satisfy a wide range of tastes. Check your local library or bookstore for this title and for others that contain low-fat, high-fiber recipes. If you are computer-savvy, the Internet can be a source of hundreds of recipes for your collection, with just a few clicks of your mouse. More information on finding recipes appears in the section called "For Further Reading," at the end of this book.

BREAKFAST

Breakfast Bran-and-Fruit Mix

> 2 cups bran flakes
> 1 cup high-fiber cereal
> ½ cup sliced or chopped nuts (almonds, walnuts, or pecans) (optional)
> ½ cup chopped dried apricots
> ½ cup chopped prunes
> ½ cup raisins

Combine bran flakes, cereal, nuts, apricots, prunes, and raisins; mix well. Store covered in an airtight container. Serve with sliced fresh fruit—apples, peaches, grapefruit sections, strawberries, bananas—and either low-fat milk or yogurt. Makes 10 servings (½ cup per serving).

Calories per ½ cup, with ½ cup low-fat milk: 219
Grams of fat per serving with milk: 7

Refrigerator Bran Muffins

1 cup vegetable oil	3 cups whole wheat flour
1 cup granulated sugar	2 teaspoons baking powder
6 eggs	2 teaspoons baking soda
⅓ cup molasses	1 teaspoon salt
3 cups low-fat milk	1 cup raisins or dates
5 cups bran	

In large bowl, beat together oil, sugar, and eggs until well mixed. Add remaining ingredients and stir until combined. Cover and refrigerate up to two weeks.

Spoon batter into paper-lined or nonstick muffin tins and bake at 425° for 15 to 20 minutes or until firm to the touch. Makes 48 medium muffins.

Tips: **Use reconstituted skim milk powder in place of milk.**

Calories: 116 per muffin
Grams of fat: 5.5 per muffin

Swiss Fruit Muesli

½ cup rolled oats
½ cup soft wheat kernels (or substitute another ½ cup of rolled oats)
½ cup raisins, chopped apricots, or prunes
2 cups low-fat yogurt or low-fat milk
Honey or maple syrup (optional)
Fresh fruit (sliced peach, pear, strawberries, banana, apple, or seedless red or green grapes)

In bowl, combine rolled oats, wheat kernels, raisins or other chopped dried fruit, nuts, and yogurt; stir until mixed. Cover and refrigerate overnight. Top with honey and fresh fruit before serving. Makes 4 servings.

Calories per serving: Approximately 240
Grams of fat per serving: 2

SALADS AND DRESSINGS

Bermuda Bean Salad

This salad keeps well in the refrigerator and is handy at a picnic or for crowd-size entertaining. The recipe can easily be halved by using 10-ounce cans of beans and half a pound each of the fresh beans, but make the same amount of marinade.

1 pound fresh wax beans
1 pound fresh green beans
1 19-ounce can red kidney beans, drained
1 19-ounce can lima or broad beans, drained
1 19-ounce can chickpeas, drained
1 19-ounce can pinto, Romano, or white kidney beans, drained
2 sweet green peppers, chopped
2 Bermuda onions, thinly sliced into rings

Marinade:

½ cup red wine vinegar
¼ cup vegetable oil
⅓ cup granulated sugar
⅓ cup packed brown sugar
1 teaspoon freshly ground pepper
½ teaspoon salt

Snap ends off fresh beans and cut into 1½-inch pieces. Cook beans in rapidly boiling water for 3 minutes; plunge into cold water until cool, then drain and pat dry. In large bowl, combine cooked beans, kidney beans, lima beans, chickpeas, green peppers, and onions.

Marinade: Combine vinegar, oil, both sugars, pepper, and salt; stir until sugars dissolve. Stir into bean mixture. Marinate in refrigerator overnight. Makes 20 servings (½ cup each).

Calories: 248 per serving
Grams fat: 4 per serving

Buttermilk Herb Dressing

    1 cup buttermilk
    ⅔ cup low-fat yogurt
    ¼ cup vegetable oil
    1 tablespoon white vinegar
    1 teaspoon dried dillweed or 3 tablespoons chopped fresh dill
    1 teaspoon Dijon mustard
    ½ teaspoon salt
    1 clove garlic, finely chopped
    Freshly ground pepper
    ⅓ cup chopped fresh parsley

In mixing bowl or large measuring cup, combine all ingredients. Using whisk or fork, mix well. Cover and refrigerate for up to 1 week. Makes 2 cups.

Calories: 18 per tablespoon
Grams of fat: 1.5 per tablespoon

Oil and Vinegar Dressing

    2 tablespoons vinegar
    ½ teaspoon Dijon mustard
    1 clove garlic, finely chopped (optional)
    Salt and freshly ground pepper
    ¼ cup vegetable, olive, or walnut oil
    3 tablespoons water
    ½ teaspoon granulated sugar (optional)

In small bowl or food processor, combine vinegar, mustard, garlic (if using), and salt and pepper to taste, and mix well. While whisking or processing, gradually add oil. Add water; taste, and add sugar if desired. Makes about ½ cup.

Calories: 51 per tablespoon
Grams of fat: 6 per tablespoon

Spinach Supper Salad

>4 cups torn spinach leaves (4 ounces)
>½ head leaf lettuce, in bite-size pieces
>2 cups alfalfa sprouts
>¼ pound mushrooms, sliced
>1 large tomato, cut in chunks
>2 scallions, chopped
>½ cup crumbled feta cheese (2 ounces)
>1 hard-cooked egg, peeled and coarsely chopped (optional)
>¼ cup dressing

In a large shallow salad bowl, toss spinach, lettuce, and alfalfa sprouts, or arrange on individual salad plates. Sprinkle mushrooms, tomato, scallions, feta cheese, and egg (if using) over top. Drizzle dressing over all. Makes 2 main-course or 6 side-salad servings.

Main-course serving (without dressing):

Calories: 230
Grams of fat: 10

SOUPS AND STEWS

Tricolor Bean Soup

2 large onions, sliced
3 cloves garlic, finely chopped
4 cups water
2 potatoes, cubed
3 carrots, cut in ¼-inch slices
1 19-ounce can pinto beans, drained (or substitute kidney beans, baby lima beans, or black-eyed peas)
1 19-ounce can kidney beans, baby lima beans, or black-eyed peas, drained
1 19-ounce can chickpeas (garbanzo beans), drained
1 teaspoon oregano
2 teaspoons basil
Salt and freshly ground pepper

In large saucepan, combine onions, garlic, water, potatoes, and carrots; bring to a boil, cover, and simmer for 20 minutes or until vegetables are tender. Add all beans, oregano, basil, and salt and pepper to taste. Simmer for 5 to 10 minutes to blend flavors. Makes 12 servings (1 cup each).

Calories: 120 per serving
Grams of fat: 1.6 per serving

Winter Vegetable Stew

    2 tablespoons vegetable oil
    4 onions, coarsely chopped
    4 large cloves garlic, finely chopped
    1 bunch leeks (3 or 4)
    4 potatoes
    4 carrots
    ½ small rutabaga (yellow turnip)
    1 sweet potato or small acorn squash (optional)
    5 cups water (preferably vegetable cooking water) or chicken
       stock
    2 teaspoons crumbled dried oregano leaves
    2 teaspoons crumbled dried thyme leaves
    2 small unpeeled zucchini, cut in chunks
    Salt and freshly ground pepper
    Chopped fresh parsley
    Grated Parmesan cheese

In large, heavy saucepan or Dutch oven, heat oil over medium heat.
Add onions and garlic; cook until tender. Discard tough green parts of
leeks; cut leeks in half lengthwise and wash under cold running water.
Cut into 3/4-inch pieces. Wash potatoes, carrots, rutabaga, and sweet
potato; cut into 1-inch cubes. (For added fiber, do not peel.) Add
vegetables (except zucchini) to saucepan as they are prepared. Stir in
water, oregano, and thyme; bring to a boil. Cover and simmer until
vegetables are tender, about 30 minutes. Stir in zucchini, and salt and
pepper to taste; simmer for 5 minutes or until all vegetables are tender,
adding more water if desired. Ladle stew into bowls and sprinkle with
parsley. Pass Parmesan separately to sprinkle over stew. Makes 6 main-
course servings.

Calories per serving: 205
Grams of fat: 4.8

ENTREES

Baked Salmon with Herbs

1 whole salmon or piece about 2½ pounds
½ cup chopped fresh parsley
2 tablespoons combination of chopped fresh herbs—dill, chives,
    chervil, basil, sage (optional)
Salt and freshly ground pepper
1 tablespoon water
1 tablespoon lemon juice
Garnish (optional): Cucumber slices, parsley, dill, or watercress

Place salmon on foil; measure thickness at thickest part. Sprinkle
parsley, herbs, and salt and pepper (to taste) inside cavity. Mix water
with lemon juice and sprinkle over outside of salmon. Fold foil over
and seal. Place wrapped salmon on baking sheet and bake in 450° oven
for 10 minutes for every 1 inch of thickness of fish, plus an additional
10 minutes cooking time because it's wrapped in foil (35 to 40 minutes
total cooking time), or until salmon is opaque. Unwrap and discard
skin; most of it should stick to foil. Place salmon on warmed platter.
Garnish with cucumber, parsley, dill, or watercress (if using).
Alternatively, arrange cooked vegetables on platter with salmon. Serve
warm with lemon wedges.

   To serve cold: While salmon is still warm, discard skin and scrape
off any dark fat. Brush salmon lightly with oil and cover with foil.
Refrigerate until serving time. Makes about 4 servings.

Calories: 391 per serving
Grams of fat: 16 per serving

Chicken Dijon

6 chicken breasts	⅓ cup low-fat yogurt
Salt and freshly ground pepper	½ cup fine fresh bread crumbs
¼ cup Dijon mustard	1 teaspoon thyme

Remove skin from chicken breasts. Sprinkle them lightly with salt and
pepper. Mix mustard into yogurt. In another bowl, mix bread crumbs,

thyme, ½ teaspoon salt, and ¼ teaspoon pepper. Spread each piece of chicken with mustard mixture, then roll in bread-crumb mixture. Place chicken in single layer on lightly greased baking sheet. Bake in 350°F oven for 45 to 50 minutes for bone-in chicken, 30 to 35 minutes for boneless, or until golden brown and meat is no longer pink inside. Makes 6 servings.

Calories: 190 per serving (241 with skin on)
Grams of fat: 3.9 per serving (8.4 with skin on)

Creamy Pasta with Broccoli, Cauliflower, and Mushrooms

1 small bunch broccoli, trimmed and cut in florets
1 small head cauliflower, trimmed and cut in florets
2 tablespoons olive oil or vegetable oil
3 cloves garlic, finely chopped
2½ cups thickly sliced mushrooms
2½ cups whole wheat noodles, egg noodles, or spaghetti
   (about 4 ounces)
1 cup low-fat small-curd cottage cheese
½ cup low-fat milk
¼ cup low-fat sour cream
¼ cup grated Parmesan cheese
Salt and cayenne pepper

In large pot of boiling water, cook cauliflower and broccoli until tender-crisp, about 5 minutes. With slotted spoon, remove vegetables and save the liquid for cooking the pasta. In large skillet, heat oil; sauté garlic and mushrooms for about 5 minutes. Stir in broccoli and cauliflower; sauté for 2 to 3 minutes longer. Set aside. Meanwhile, in reserved boiling vegetable liquid, cook pasta, adding water if necessary, until al dente (tender but firm), about 8 to 10 minutes; drain. In food processor, combine cottage cheese, milk, sour cream, and Parmesan. Pour over broccoli mixture; add drained pasta and toss until mixed. Season with salt and cayenne pepper to taste. Serve immediately. Makes about 8 servings.

Calories: 301 per serving
Grams of fat: 5 per serving

Fettuccine with Fresh Tomatoes and Basil

> 6 ounces fettuccine noodles or 2 cups dried medium egg noodles
> *(for maximum fiber, use whole wheat noodles)*
> 2 tablespoons olive oil
> 2 cloves garlic, finely chopped
> 4 tomatoes, diced
> ½ teaspoon dried basil or 2 tablespoons chopped fresh
> Pinch granulated sugar
> ¼ cup chopped fresh parsley
> Salt and freshly ground pepper
> 2 tablespoons grated Parmesan cheese

In large pot of boiling water, cook noodles until al dente (tender but firm). Meanwhile, in heavy skillet, heat oil over medium heat; stir in garlic, tomatoes, basil, and sugar, and cook for 5 minutes, stirring occasionally. Add parsley, and salt and pepper to taste. (If sauce is too thick, add a few spoonfuls of pasta cooking liquid.) Drain noodles. Toss with tomato mixture and Parmesan. Pass extra Parmesan. Makes two main-course servings, four appetizer or side-dish servings.

> **Calories per main-course serving: 425**
> **Grams of fat per main-course serving: 14**

Marinated Flank Steak

> 1 pound flank steak
> ¼ cup soy sauce
> ¼ cup vegetable oil
> 2 tablespoons vinegar
> 2 tablespoons sugar or honey
> 1 tablespoon peeled and grated fresh ginger root or 1 teaspoon
>   ground ginger

Score one side of the steak by making shallow cuts in a crisscross pattern. Place meat in a shallow dish or plastic bag. Combine soy sauce, oil, vinegar, sugar, and ginger; pour over meat. Cover, and refrigerate for 1 to 3 days, or let stand at room temperature for up to 3 hours. Remove meat from marinade and broil for 4 to 5 minutes on each side. Slice thinly on an angle, across the grain. Serve hot or cold. Makes 4 servings.

Calories: 200 per serving
Grams of fat: 9 per serving

Old-Fashioned Meat Loaf

> 1 pound lean ground beef
> 1 large onion, finely chopped
> ¼ cup natural bran
> 1 slice whole wheat bread, crumbed
> ½ teaspoon thyme
> ½ teaspoon salt
> Dash Worcestershire sauce
> Freshly ground pepper
> 1 cup tomato juice or tomato sauce
> 1 egg, lightly beaten
> 1 tablespoon chopped fresh herbs — thyme, rosemary, savory,
>   sage (optional)

In mixing bowl, combine beef, onion, bran, bread crumbs, thyme, salt, Worcestershire, and pepper to taste. Stir in tomato juice, egg, and herbs (if using); mix lightly. Turn into 9 × 5-inch loaf pan or baking dish. Bake in 350°F oven for 45 minutes, or until brown and firm to the touch. Remove from oven; pour off fat. Makes 5 servings.

Calories: 186 per serving (lean ground beef); 267 (regular ground beef)
Grams of fat: 9.5 (lean); 17 (regular)

Sole Filets with Lemon and Parsley

1 pound sole filets (or substitute cod, snapper, or perch)
Salt and freshly ground pepper
2 teaspoons butter, melted
2 tablespoons chopped fresh parsley
1 tablespoon lemon juice

Place filets in lightly oiled baking dish just large enough to hold them in single layer. Sprinkle with salt and pepper to taste. Combine butter, parsley, and lemon juice. Drizzle over fish. Bake, uncovered, in 450°F oven for 8 to 10 minutes (10 minutes per inch thickness for fresh fish) or until fish is opaque and flakes easily. To microwave: Cover with plastic wrap and turn back corner to vent for steam; microwave on high for 3½ to 4½ minutes. Makes 4 servings.

Calories: 117 per serving
Grams of fat: 7 per serving

VEGETABLES

Broccoli and Sweet Pepper Stir-Fry

1 bunch broccoli (about
   1 pound)
1 sweet red pepper
1 sweet yellow pepper
1 tablespoon vegetable oil

1 onion, chopped
1 teaspoon grated fresh
   ginger root
¼ cup chicken stock
2 teaspoons soy sauce

Peel tough broccoli stems. Cut stems and florets into pieces about 1½ inches long. Blanch in large pot of boiling water for 2 to 3 minutes or until bright green and tender-crisp; drain, cool under cold running water, and dry on paper towels. Seed peppers and cut into thin strips.

(This can be done in advance.) In large, heavy skillet or wok, heat oil over medium heat. Add onion and ginger; stir-fry for 1 minute. Add peppers and stir-fry for 2 to 3 minutes, adding chicken stock when necessary to prevent sticking or scorching. Add broccoli; stir-fry until heated through; sprinkle with soy sauce. Serve immediately. Makes 8 servings.

Calories: 40 per serving
Grams of fat: 2 per serving

Mashed Potatoes with Onions

6 potatoes*
2 teaspoons butter
2 onions, finely chopped
1 tablespoon water
½ cup low-fat milk
Salt and pepper

*For maximum fiber, do not peel

Peel potatoes and cut into quarters. Cook potatoes in boiling water until tender, about 20 minutes. Meanwhile, in heavy skillet, melt butter; add onions and water and cook over medium-low heat, stirring occasionally, until onions are tender, 10 to 15 minutes, reducing the heat if necessary so onions don't brown. Drain potatoes and return pan to stove; heat over low heat for 1 to 2 minutes, shaking pan to dry potatoes. Mash potatoes with half of the milk, adding remaining milk to taste (amount of milk needed will vary, depending on size and kind of potatoes). Stir in onions, add salt and pepper to taste. Makes 6 servings.

Calories: 123 per serving
Grams of fat: 2

Tarragon Carrots

4 large carrots, thinly sliced
(2 cups)
2 small onions, thinly
sliced
1 teaspoon tarragon

2 tablespoons water
Salt and freshly ground
pepper
2 teaspoons butter

Lightly oil a large sheet of foil or a 6-cup microwave dish. On foil or in dish, place carrots and onion; sprinkle with tarragon, water, and pepper to taste. Wrap tightly or cover. Cook in 350°F oven for 30 minutes, or microwave on high for 10 to 12 minutes, or until tender. Stir in butter and salt to taste. Makes 4 servings.

Calories: 37 per serving
Grams of fat: 2 per serving

BREAD

Wheat Germ Crisp Cookies

1¼ cups whole wheat flour
1 cup wheat germ
1 teaspoon cinnamon
¼ teaspoon ground cloves
¼ teaspoon salt
½ cup butter or margarine

½ cup packed brown sugar
1 egg
1 teaspoon vanilla
2 tablespoons granulated
sugar

In bowl, combine flour, wheat germ, cinnamon, cloves, and salt; mix well. In another large bowl, cream butter and brown sugar thoroughly; beat in egg and vanilla. Add mixed dry ingredients to creamed mixture and mix well. Divide dough in half. On lightly floured counter, roll each half ⅛ inch thick. Cut with 2½-inch round cutter. Place on ungreased baking sheets. Sprinkle with granulated sugar. Bake in 350°F oven for 8 to 10 minutes or until lightly browned. Let cool until firm, then remove from baking sheets. Makes 36 cookies.

Calories: 57 per cookie
Grams of fat: 3 per cookie

Whole Wheat Irish Soda Bread

    3 cups whole wheat flour
    1 cup all-purpose flour
    2 tablespoons granulated sugar
    2 teaspoons baking powder
    1½ teaspoons baking soda
    1 teaspoon salt
    2 tablespoons butter
    1¾ cups buttermilk (or 1¾ cups low-fat milk, plus 2 tablespoons
      vinegar)

Combine flours, sugar, baking powder, baking soda, and salt. With pastry blender or two knives, cut in butter until crumbly. Add buttermilk and stir to make a soft dough. Turn out onto lightly floured counter and knead about 10 times, until smooth. Place dough on greased baking sheet; flatten into circle about 2½ inches thick. Cut a large "X" about ¼ inch deep on top. Bake in 350°F oven for 1 hour or until toothpick inserted in center comes out clean. Makes 1 loaf (about 16 slices).

    Calories: 143 per slice
    Grams of fat: 1.7 per slice

Whole Wheat Raisin Scones

3 tablespoons granulated
 sugar
1 cup all-purpose flour
1 cup whole wheat flour
1 tablespoon baking powder
1½ teaspoons cinnamon

½ teaspoon nutmeg
½ teaspoon salt
⅓ cup butter or margarine
2 eggs, lightly beaten
⅓ cup low-fat milk
½ cup raisins

Reserve 1 teaspoon of the sugar. In mixing bowl, combine remaining sugar, both flours, baking powder, cinnamon, nutmeg, and salt. With pastry blender or two knives, cut in butter until mixture resembles coarse crumbs. Reserve 1 tablespoon of the beaten eggs. Stir remaining eggs, milk, and raisins into flour mixture and mix lightly. Turn out onto lightly floured counter and knead about 5 times. Pat into a circle about ¾ inch thick. Cut into 12 wedges and place slightly apart on greased baking sheet. Brush reserved beaten egg over each wedge; sprinkle with reserved sugar. Bake in 425°F oven for 18 to 20 minutes or until browned. Serve warm. Makes 12 scones.

Calories: 146 per serving
Grams fat: 5 per serving
[Source: ACS]

DESSERTS

Almond-Apricot Squares

¾ cup packed dried apricots
½ cup butter
1¼ cups whole wheat flour
¾ cup chopped almonds
¾ cup granulated sugar

¼ cup bran or wheat germ
½ teaspoon cinnamon
2 eggs
½ teaspoon almond extract
½ teaspoon baking powder
½ teaspoon salt

In small saucepan, combine apricots with enough water to cover. Cover and bring to a boil; reduce heat and simmer for 20 minutes. Drain, let cool. Chop apricots finely; set aside. In mixing bowl, cut butter into 1 cup flour. Mix in ¼ cup of the almonds, ¼ cup of the sugar, bran, and cinnamon. Press half of this mixture into greased 8-inch-square baking pan. In another mixing bowl, beat remaining ½ cup sugar with eggs and almond extract. Beat in baking powder, salt, apricots, remaining ¼ cup flour, and remaining ½ cup almonds. Pour over layer in pan. Sprinkle with remaining flour-bran mixture. Bake in 350°F oven for 40 minutes. Let cool, then cut into squares. Makes about 18 pieces.

Calories: 77 per square
Grams of fat: 4 per square

Cinnamon Coffee Cake

1 cup low-fat yogurt
1 teaspoon baking soda
¼ cup butter or margarine
1 cup lightly packed brown sugar
1 egg
1 teaspoon vanilla
1½ cups all-purpose flour
2 teaspoons baking powder

Topping:

½ cup lightly packed brown sugar
1 tablespoon cinnamon

Grease and flour a bundt pan or 9-inch-square baking pan. In small bowl, combine yogurt and baking soda; mix well and set aside. (Yogurt mixture will increase in volume.) In large mixing bowl, beat butter with sugar until well mixed. Add egg and vanilla; beat well, about 2 minutes. Sift together flour and baking powder; add to butter mixture alternately with yogurt mixture.

Topping: Combine sugar and cinnamon; mix well. Spread half the batter in prepared pan. Sprinkle with half the topping. Cover with remaining batter and sprinkle with remaining topping. Bake in 350°F oven for 45 minutes or until toothpick inserted in center comes out clean. Let cool for 10 to 15 minutes in pan, then invert onto wire rack. Makes 12 servings.

Calories per serving: 170
Grams fat per serving: 4

Clafouti (French Baked-Fruit Custard)

    4 cups fresh apricots (or substitute cherries, plums, or peaches)
    1 tablespoon butter
    6 tablespoons granulated sugar
    3 eggs
    1¾ cups low-fat milk
    ⅔ cup all-purpose flour
    1 teaspoon grated lemon rind
    ½ teaspoon cinnamon
    2 teaspoons vanilla
    Pinch salt
    Confectioners' sugar

Halve apricots, then pit them. Grease an 11-inch glass pie plate or large quiche dish with the butter. Sprinkle with 1 tablespoon of the granulated sugar. Arrange apricots, cut side down, in dish and sprinkle with 2 tablespoons of the granulated sugar. In blender or food processor, combine remaining sugar, eggs, milk, flour, lemon rind, cinnamon, vanilla, and salt; process until smooth. Alternatively, beat remaining sugar with eggs; add remaining ingredients and beat until smooth. Pour mixture evenly over fruit. Bake in 375°F oven for 50 to 60 minutes or until top is browned and filling is set. Just before serving, sift confectioners' sugar over top. Serve warm or cold. Makes 6 to 8 servings.

    Calories: 160–210 (depending on size of serving)
    Grams of fat: 4.4–58 (depending on size of serving)

Poached Pears with Chocolate Sauce

  3 cups water
  ½ cup granulated sugar
  Grated rind and juice of 1 lemon
  1 vanilla bean and/or cinnamon stick
  4 pears
  ¼ cup easy chocolate sauce

Easy chocolate sauce:

  1 cup cocoa
  ¾ cup granulated sugar
  ¾ cup water
  ½ cup corn syrup
  1 teaspoon vanilla

In large saucepan, combine water, sugar, lemon rind, lemon juice, vanilla bean and/or cinnamon stick. Bring to a boil, stirring until sugar is dissolved. Peel, halve, and core pears. Add to boiling syrup. (Pears should be covered in liquid; if not, double the amount of poaching liquid, or poach in batches.) Reduce heat to medium-low and simmer gently for 15 to 20 minutes or until pears are almost tender. (Time will vary, depending on ripeness and type of pear; remember, pears will continue to cook while cooling.) Remove from heat and let cool in liquid. Drain pears thoroughly and pat dry with paper towels. Arrange on individual plates. Drizzle with sauce. Serve at room temperature. Makes 4 large servings or 8 small.

  Sauce: In saucepan, combine cocoa and sugar. Whisk in water and corn syrup. Bring to a full boil over medium heat; boil for 2 minutes, stirring constantly. Remove from heat and stir in vanilla. Let cool (sauce will thicken upon cooling). Cover and store in refrigerator. Makes 2 cups sauce.

  Calories: 200 per small serving
  Grams of fat: 1.1 per small serving

Prune Cake

1½ cups prunes
1½ cups water
¾ cup packed brown sugar
⅓ cup granulated sugar
1 cup low-fat yogurt
2 eggs

1½ cups all-purpose flour
1 cup whole wheat flour
2 teaspoons baking powder
½ teaspoon baking soda
1 teaspoon cinnamon
½ teaspoon salt

In saucepan, combine prunes and water; bring to a boil and simmer for 1 minute. Cover and let stand until cool; drain. Remove pits and chop prunes (you should have about 1½ cups); set aside. In mixing bowl, combine sugars and yogurt; beat until smooth. Add eggs and beat until well mixed. Add flours, baking powder, baking soda, cinnamon, and salt; beat well. Stir in prunes. Pour into lightly greased and floured 12 × 8-inch baking pan. Bake in 375°F oven for 30 minutes or until toothpick inserted in center comes out clean. Makes 18 servings.

Calories: 140 per serving
Grams of fat: 1.25 per serving

Rhubarb Crumb Pie

Pastry:

¾ cup all-purpose flour
½ cup whole wheat flour
½ teaspoon salt
3 tablespoons butter or
    margarine
3 tablespoons ice water

Filling:

1 cup granulated sugar
¼ cup all-purpose flour
1 teaspoon grated orange or
    lemon rind
1 egg, well beaten
5 cups sliced fresh or frozen
    (thawed) rhubarb, cut
    into ½-inch pieces

Topping:

⅓ cup packed brown sugar
3 tablespoons rolled oats
3 tablespoons powdered skim milk (optional)
3 tablespoons whole wheat flour
1 teaspoon cinnamon
2 tablespoons butter

Pastry: In mixing bowl, combine flours and salt. With pastry blender or two knives, cut in butter until mixture is crumbly. Sprinkle water over mixture and toss with a fork to mix. Press onto bottom and up sides of a 9-inch pie plate. (For a simpler recipe, purchase a frozen pie shell.)

Filling: Combine sugar, flour, and grated orange rind; mix well. In another bowl, mix egg and rhubarb; add sugar mixture and stir to mix.

Topping: In bowl, combine sugar, rolled oats, powdered milk (if using), flour, and cinnamon. Cut in butter until mixture is crumbly.

Spoon rhubarb filling into pie shell. Sprinkle topping over filling. Bake in 400°F oven for 50 to 60 minutes or until top is golden brown and rhubarb is tender. To prevent top from becoming too brown, cover lightly with foil after 30 minutes of baking. Makes 8 servings.

Calories: 285 per serving
Grams of fat: 8 per serving

Chapter 12

Living with Colorectal Cancer

Over the years, as you cope with colorectal cancer, you and your loved ones will experience a range of strong, and often conflicting, feelings: hope and despair; fear and courage; anger and humor. For some people, the disease becomes the central focus, the event around which everything else is organized. Others refuse to let cancer take control of their lives. There is no right way or wrong way. Everyone has a different style of coping with the situation.

In surgical and medical treatment for colorectal cancer, the focus is on removing the tumor and all cancerous cells from your body. But these methods do not treat the overwhelming emotions that are bound to emerge during the course of your illness. It is important to be aware of these feelings; it is equally important to know that people and resources are available to help you manage them. This chapter briefly discusses some of the emotional concerns, as well as some solutions. It also touches on some practical matters, such as managing a colostomy and dealing with financial issues. For more information, contact the organizations listed in the "Resources" section at the back of this book.

COPING WITH A COLOSTOMY

For many people who undergo surgery for colorectal cancer, the possibility that they will have to have a colostomy is the greatest concern. A colostomy is a surgical procedure in which part of the colon is brought through an opening in the abdominal wall. A similar procedure, called an ileostomy, brings the end of the ileum (the lowest end of the small intestine) through the abdominal wall. These procedures create an artificial opening, or *stoma*, through which feces and gas can exit the body. The fecal material is collected in a bag or pouch attached to the skin.

For most patients, a colostomy is only temporary. It can be reversed after the colon has had time to rest. The time needed for healing ranges from a few weeks to a year or more. At the end of that time, normal bowel activity (including normal defecation) returns. In a small proportion of cases, especially those involving surgery in the lower part of the rectum, the organ no longer functions and the colostomy must remain permanently in place. The medical term for people with a colostomy or an ileostomy is *ostomates*.

As you learned in Chapter 2, the main functions of the colon are to absorb water from fecal material and move the stool along until it can be eliminated through the anus. Because most of the nutrients from food are absorbed in the small intestine, colectomy or colostomy will not significantly affect the nourishment you get from your meals.

The nature of the material that passes through an ostomy depends on how much of the colon, and which section, is removed during surgery. A right hemicolectomy (removing the right side of the colon) usually does not require an ileostomy. Usually, an anastomos is made to connect the ileum to the left side of the colon.

Cancer in the transverse colon also may mean the loss of a large portion of the colon. Less colon remains to absorb water, so the material is usually more fluid, and discharge through the stoma occurs more frequently. In contrast, removal of the descending or the sigmoid colon means that the material remains in the intestine longer, so it tends to be firmer and it is expelled at more regular intervals.

The location of the stoma also depends on the part of the colon affected by surgery. An ileostomy appears on the right side of the abdomen, a little to the right of and a little below the navel (Figure 12.1).

If the surgery removes the lower part of the descending colon, the stoma will appear on the left side of the abdomen next to the navel (Figure 12.2A). Surgery to remove the sigmoid colon produces a stoma a few inches lower (Figure 12.2B). Sigmoid colostomies are the most frequently performed type of colostomy.

A colostomy may result in two openings. One stoma discharges feces from the active appear portion of the colon; the other discharges mucus from the "resting" colon (the lower portion that is still alive but no longer processes feces). When the two openings are close enough to appear as one, this is called a loop colostomy (Figure 12.3). When they are farther apart, they form two distinct openings; this is known as a double-barrel colostomy (Figure 12.4). (Operations involving the transverse colon result in a stoma on the right side above the navel.)

If you have a colostomy, you must learn to take special care of your body so as to reduce the risk of complications. Prior to colorectal surgery, the physician and a nurse specializing in the care of ostomies (known as an enterostomal therapy nurse, or ET nurse) will discuss the situation with you. You may not require a colostomy at all, but you need to be prepared in case you wake up after the operation and find that one has been made.

In the first days after the procedure, the stoma may appear quite large. The tissue will be swollen or bruised, and may be deep red in color. There may be stitches. The tissue visible in the stoma is a mucous membrane somewhat like the lining of the cheek. It does not contain muscle, however, so it cannot be shut or squeezed tight, as the anus can. That's why there is no control over when feces are discharged, and why the colostomy bag usually must be worn at all times. Over the next six to eight weeks, the size of the stoma will gradually shrink, and its color will change to a lighter red or pink.

Following surgery, the resting colon continues to produce mucus. Some of this material exits through the colostomy, and the rest is passed through the anus. This is normal.

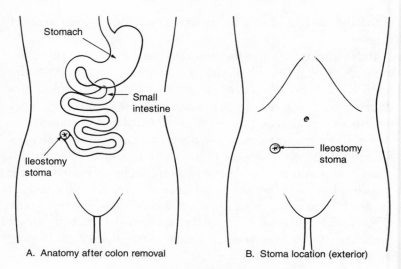

A. Anatomy after colon removal

B. Stoma location (exterior)

Figure 12.1: Ileostomy.

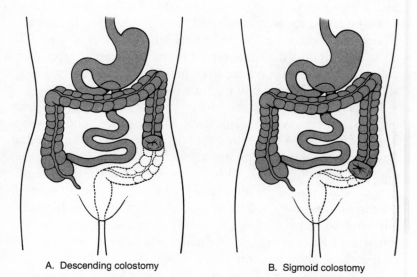

A. Descending colostomy

B. Sigmoid colostomy

Figure 12.2: Stoma locations—left side.

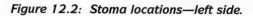

As mentioned earlier, the discharge from an ileostomy or a transverse colostomy is very liquid. It also contains digestive enzymes, which can be irritating to the skin. A drainable pouch is worn over these openings to collect the discharge and protect the skin from irritation.

Descending or sigmoid colostomies produce firmer stool that does not contain enzymes and is less irritating. Elimination may occur at regular, predictable intervals, usually after a considerable quantity of stool has collected. In some cases, but not all, ostomates who had regular bowel movements prior to surgery discover they can "train" the colostomy to produce a movement reflexively. Sometimes, though, use of a mild stimulant, such as coffee or a laxative, may be needed. Two or three days may elapse between movements. To be safe, ostomates usually wear a lightweight, disposable pouch all the time to collect any accidental discharge.

Caring for a colostomy is not difficult, but it does require learning, practice, the right materials, and a positive attitude. In the early phase of a colostomy, stools will be unpredictable in consistency and in frequency. Gradually, however, a pattern will be established. Working with your doctor and your ET nurse, you will discover a strategy for catching movements in time to avoid surprises and embarrassment.

Several types of appliances are available. Within a short time, you and your caregivers will identify the one that is right for you. Advances in technology have led to pouches that are small and inconspicuous and that help to control odor. Some pouches have openings at the bottom for easy emptying; others are closed and are removed when filled. Another kind has a "face plate" that remains attached to the abdomen while the pouch is removed, cleaned, and replaced. If you gain or lose weight, you may need to be fitted with a different type of pouch to make sure the opening is completely covered.

Some ostomates do not wear a collection pouch regularly. Instead, they control release of the material by irrigating the

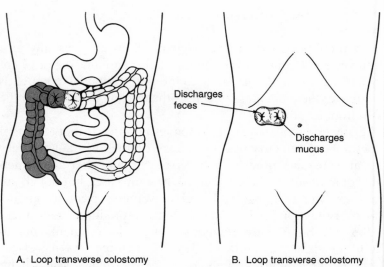

A. Loop transverse colostomy
(interior).

B. Loop transverse colostomy
(exterior).

Figure 12.3: Loop colostomy: two stomas close together.

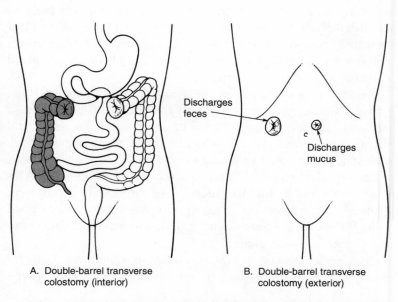

A. Double-barrel transverse
colostomy (interior)

B. Double-barrel transverse
colostomy (exterior)

Figure 12.4: Double-barrel colostomy: two separate stomas.

colostomy (that is, by performing a kind of enema). The ET nurse will explain how to perform an irrigation.

Gas and odor are part of the digestive process and cannot be prevented. However, your caregivers will teach you ways to minimize and control these problems. For example, to reduce gas, eat at a leisurely pace, chew food well with your mouth closed, and use chewing gum or carbonated drinks in moderation. Avoid gas-producing foods, such as cucumbers, cabbage, broccoli, mushrooms, onions, and beans. If you are lactose intolerant (that is, you lack an enzyme you need to digest dairy products properly), also avoid milk and cheese. These same foods can also increase odor, as can certain medications and vitamins. Special oral deodorants and odor-proof, single-use pouches are available.

By emptying the appliance several times a day, you reduce the risk of leaks and telltale bulges under your clothes. Most people use a fresh appliance every one to three days. Using a correctly fitted appliance reduces the risk of skin irritation.

If the stoma behaves predictably and a pouch is not worn, the stoma can be covered with tissue or gauze covered with plastic wrap and held in place with tape. Plastic stoma caps are also available.

There is no such thing as a "colostomy diet," but the food you eat can have some effect on a colostomy. Generally, you can eat the same foods you enjoyed prior to your operation. Some people with a descending or sigmoid colostomy find that eating certain foods at specific intervals can trigger a movement at predictable (and more convenient) times. This allows them to avoid wearing a pouch unless a movement is anticipated. Various foods can also make movements more or less liquid. As a rule, however, it is not a good idea to try to control discharge through a transverse colostomy with special diets, medications, enemas, or irrigations. Do not use laxatives unless your caregivers advise you to do so.

Next to skin irritation, the most common problem with colostomies is herniation, or bulging of the skin around the stoma. This makes irrigation difficult, blocks the opening, and can lead to prolapse, in which part of the bowel protrudes through the opening. Careful placement of the stoma during surgery minimizes this risk. Over time, the stoma may become stiff and narrow (stenotic), due to continued irrigation injury or reduced blood supply. A minor operation can usually correct the problem. Rupture or perforation of the colon is a risk if the irrigation catheter is inserted incorrectly.

The thought of a colostomy is disturbing, but remember that, after adjusting to the situation, most ostomates are able to live normal, active lives. People with colostomies can function at work (although they should avoid heavy lifting). A colostomy need not be a barrier to travel, exercise, or participation in noncontact sports. There is no reason to avoid socializing; many of your friends will never know that you have a colostomy unless you tell them. A normal sex life is still possible, although the couple needs to discuss openly and honestly their feelings about the changes in the ostomate's body.

SUPPORT GROUPS

There is safety, and there is strength, in numbers. The people most likely to understand what you're going through are those who are going through it themselves. That's where a support group comes in.

Support groups offer you a chance to meet with other people with cancer, and their loved ones, to discuss common problems and explore new solutions. In the past few decades, support groups have proved to be one of the most valuable assets for cancer recovery. Knowing that you are not alone, that other people have wrestled with—and have overcome—the same challenges that you face is deeply reassuring. Support groups are a source of understanding, insight, compassion, and love.

Although a support group can be "therapeutic"—that is, taking part can improve your sense of wellness and your satisfaction with living—its goals and methods differ from those of a therapy group, as I'll discuss in a moment.

Different types of support groups are available, depending on your needs. Groups may meet in hospitals, community centers, churches or synagogues, or private homes. Most group meetings are available free of charge (although sometimes donations are accepted to defray expenses).

Open-ended groups meet regularly for an unlimited period of time. People can "drop in," attending whenever they feel that doing so would be of benefit, and they can withdraw when they no longer wish to take part. Topics addressed at these meetings can cover everything from how to find a good doctor to coping with the physical and emotional side effects of treatment. Some open-ended groups have been in existence for years. *Time-limited groups* hold meetings with the same members each time, and they meet for a certain designated period, such as three months.

The leadership of groups varies. A group leader might be a medical professional, a trained facilitator such as a social worker, a person recovering from cancer, or some combination of these individuals. In meetings, groups discuss the latest treatments, strategies for coping with physical and emotional concerns, and other related topics. The presence of a doctor or nurse ensures that any medical information presented will be accurate and useful. Other groups are created and managed entirely by the members themselves. These groups offer strong emotional support and a forum for discussing deeply personal concerns. Unless a medical professional is present, such groups are not intended to be a source of accurate medical information.

Membership depends on the goals the group wishes to achieve. Some groups include only people who have colorectal cancer; others might include people with any form of cancer. Some groups welcome spouses or other close family members; others are designed specifically for couples, or for men only or women only, or for people in a certain age bracket.

Some groups address specific problems that each of the members has in common, such as coping with colostomies or dealing with family responses. Time-limited groups are more likely to focus on such issues. In some groups, the purpose is basically educational. Guest speakers present talks on topics of interest, which the members might then discuss. Other groups are less structured; members can talk about anything that concerns them at that particular time. Topics might range from dealing with upset family members to addressing problems in the workplace. Some groups may be more social in nature, providing a place for people who are coping with a common problem to gather and to celebrate another day of survival. Many people who meet in groups become close friends.

Not every person with cancer will feel like joining a support group. Some may be uncomfortable talking about medical problems or emotional issues with strangers. Understandably, others would rather spend their time thinking about anything *but* their disease. For these individuals, individual counseling or therapy may be more beneficial.

Another resource is a peer counselor, a cancer survivor who volunteers time to meet with other people who have the disease, talk about problems, and help find solutions. Some peer counselors work with support groups; others are available for one-on-one sessions. If you don't think you'd be comfortable in a group, you may prefer to talk privately with a peer counselor.

For most people, group participation becomes a vital part of their survival strategy. They discover that being a group member helps them and provides an opportunity for them to help others. Many find that offering support and guidance to new members can be among their most rewarding and meaningful experiences.

To find out about the support groups and peer counseling programs available in your area, ask your doctor, nurse, social worker, or hospital patient advocate. You can also contact the American Cancer Society (1–800-ACS-2345; http://www.cancer.org), the Cancer Information Service of the National Cancer Institute

(1–800-4CANCER; http://www.cancernet.nci.nih.gov), or other organizations listed in the "Resources" section at the back of this book.

GROUP THERAPY

As support groups have shown, a lot of good can come from being in a room full of people who are working to overcome a shared problem. Group therapy accomplishes similar goals. The main difference is that a therapy group is facilitated by one or more trained professionals, usually a psychologist, psychiatrist, or social worker, and a support group is usually conducted by the members themselves (often in conjunction with a professional).

In therapy, the group leader has the responsibility for organizing the sessions, establishing rules for how discussions will be conducted, and deciding what topics will be addressed. Often, the leader will assign tasks or therapeutic exercises designed to help resolve participants' problems. Support groups are usually less structured and more open-ended. Members are often encouraged to speak about whatever is on their mind, whether it is related directly to cancer or not. In a therapy group, the leader guides the discussion to stay focused on the specific problem the participants share in common.

Therapy groups typically involve eight to ten people. Often, spouses or family members are included. Meetings might be held once or twice a week for an hour. Support groups are usually free of charge, but group therapy involves a fee.

INDIVIDUAL, MARITAL, AND FAMILY COUNSELING

Coping with a serious and lifelong illness such as colorectal cancer puts tremendous strain on all your important relationships. Some couples and their families find that facing this mutual challenge makes them grow closer to one another. In other families, the burden of coping with treatment, the emotional turmoil of watching a loved one suffer, and the disruption in daily life takes a toll on everyone in the household. Many people find it hard to communicate their feelings, especially their fear of pain and death. Spouses may fear being left alone; young children may worry about being abandoned. In an effort to keep up each other's spirits and to not upset anyone, families may avoid frank and open discussions of unpleasant subjects. Worries about money and the future can be draining. Cancer and its treatment can cause fatigue, depression, and withdrawal from social life; these problems affect not only the person with the disease but everyone in the household.

Under such circumstances, married couples or other partners may find it very hard to maintain emotional closeness and physical intimacy. Sexual desire may dwindle or disappear. Naturally, it is hard to think about sexual activity when all of your energy is focused mainly on surviving the disease. The symptoms of cancer and the side effects of treatment can diminish desire even further. The presence of a colostomy can pose a further barrier to intimacy. Misunderstandings are common. One partner may avoid initiating sexual contact out of concern for the other, but this can send a message that the spouse is undesirable or unloved. Some people have the totally false notion that sexual intercourse can transmit cancer to the partner.

Counseling can potentially help you address all of these circumstances. Sessions with a trained professional can help bring a couple's or a family's problems into the open and can point the way toward solutions. Counselors don't tell people what they should do. Instead, they help them identify problems, discover solutions, and develop the communication and relationship skills they need to put those solutions into action. Families who take advantage of counseling may learn new ways to talk to each other, to express their needs more clearly, and to avoid pressing the "hot buttons" that can disrupt communication.

Sexuality may be the only problem, or the primary problem, a couple is dealing with. Sexual counseling can zero in on this issue. Couples might benefit by learning how to talk about the situation and by discovering solutions to impotence or other problems that may result from cancer therapy. Counselors can provide practical advice on how to manage an ostomy during intercourse. Not everyone will need or will benefit from counseling. Families that already have good communication skills and have "learned how to fight" can often find ways to solve their own problems. For others, however, working with a counselor may speed up the process of finding solutions. If one partner or family member refuses to take part in counseling, the other members of the family may still benefit. Individual sessions can also be valuable.

SPIRITUAL COUNSELING

For many people, a diagnosis of cancer triggers a deep reexamination of the value and meaning of their lives. Wondering what they have done to deserve cancer as a punishment, some begin to feel angry or hopeless. Others see their disease as a challenge from God, and they resolve to make every remaining minute count. Feelings of guilt, anger, or despair can be overwhelming.

Many cancer patients—even those who do not think of themselves as religious—will seek spiritual guidance as part of their process of coping with their disease. Many churches, synagogues, mosques, and hospitals have staff or peer counselors whose role is to meet with patients and their families and talk about such issues. Comfort may come in the form of prayers for healing, or insightful discussion about the meaning of the disease and of life. Some religious organizations can provide practical help, ranging from financial support to pay for treatment to volunteers who drive patients to their medical appointments.

In cases involving advanced or recurring cancer, people are tempted to give up on medical treatment and rely instead on prayer. The two options are not mutually exclusive. Receiving medical attention should not prevent prayer, and prayer should not interfere with sound medical therapy. On the contrary, prayer or other ritual practices can be a tremendous source of comfort, support, and serenity. By providing peace of mind, spiritual guidance can go a long way in relieving the suffering associated with cancer and its treatment.

Many spiritual counseling services are available at no cost. If you are seeking help in this regard, try to find a counselor who has some experience in dealing with cancer-related problems. Your doctor, clergy, or hospital representative can help.

HELP FOR DEPRESSION

Depression is a serious emotional illness that can result from drastic changes in life situations, sudden profound loss, or changes in the body. Not surprisingly, some people with cancer (but not all) also experience depression.

Depression is like a black cloud that surrounds the mind and the heart, robbing life of its joy. The disorder causes profound feelings of sadness, despair, guilt, fatigue, and hopelessness. People with depression often withdraw from family and friends. They lose interest in activities that formerly brought them pleasure. Their ability to work or to maintain relationships dwindles. Changes in their eating habits can result in significant weight loss or weight gain. Often, people with depression find it difficult to fall asleep at night, or they wake up too early in the morning. Sexual desire can disappear. Even the will to live is affected. A significant number of depressed people think about or actually attempt suicide. The risk is higher when a serious chronic disease like colorectal cancer is involved; it makes the future seem especially bleak.

Depression can be a specific symptom of cancer. The physical effects of the disease can disrupt the chemical balance in the brain, leading to disturbed moods and changes in the body's senses. Depression can also arise as a side effect of cancer treatment, especially during chemotherapy.

Depression is not the same as feeling sad or blue. Sadness is a normal—and temporary—reaction to bad news (such as a diagnosis of cancer) or to the stress of coping with a serious problem. Over the course of a few days, the sadness usually lifts. Depression, by contrast, can persist for weeks or months—or even for years. Well-meaning but misinformed people might tell a depressed person with cancer, "Just snap out it" or "Stop feeling sorry for yourself." The truth is, no one can just "snap out of" depression.

Fortunately, there are many effective treatments. Some people benefit simply by talking about their situation with understanding family and friends, with members of a support group, or with a trained counselor. For others, antidepressant medications may help, especially when combined with some form of talk therapy (also called psychotherapy). Relieving depression lowers the level of emotional turmoil, relieves feelings of helplessness and hopelessness, and increases energy level. A person can then more easily continue receiving other forms of cancer therapy. Thus, treatment for depression can indirectly improve the outcome of cancer treatment.

Antidepressants require a doctor's prescription and supervision; psychotherapy can be provided by a psychiatrist, psychologist, counselor, or other caregiver. Seeing a mental health professional does not mean you are "crazy." Quite the contrary: Getting effective help for a troubling emotional problem is a sign of strength.

DEALING WITH PROBLEMS ON THE JOB

If you work, coping with colorectal cancer in the years ahead can have an impact on your job or your career. Most people are able to return to work after a period of recovery from colorectal surgery, if that's their choice. Some people need a year of recuperation before they feel able to work full time. Others rebound more quickly.

Some employers are tolerant and understanding of a cancer survivor's special needs. They are willing to work out flexible schedules to permit time off for doctor's visits and procedures. It may be possible to change assignments within the company— temporarily, if need be—to reduce physical or emotional stress.

For some patients, though, problems are bound to arise. Companies may be reluctant to hire cancer survivors or consider them for promotions. They may worry about the employee's productivity or job attendance. Such fears are usually groundless. Research shows that cancer survivors are just as productive as other workers and, on average, they take no more time off from work than other employees.

Dealing with coworkers can also pose challenges. Many people are frightened by cancer because they don't understand the disease. Some assume that cancer is always fatal, or that it is contagious, or that it makes you less able to do your job. None of those myths is true, but it may take a little education to help coworkers realize that they are myths. If you are managing a colostomy, you must be prepared for workplace reactions ranging from disgust to curiosity, compassion, and support. A frank and open discussion often allays fears and corrects misunderstandings. Depending on your needs and circumstances, you may want to discuss your condition at a departmental meeting. Or, you might consider asking the personnel manager, medical officer, union leader, or other executive to sponsor an educational presentation by a doctor or nurse.

Unfortunately, given human nature, problems in the workplace may still arise. About one out of four cancer survivors who return to work experiences some type of job discrimination. Sometimes, discussing the problem with the boss or with coworkers can resolve the issue, but it may be necessary to involve a manager, shop steward, personnel representative, or union official.

You may also be protected by state or federal laws. To learn more, contact your local American Cancer Society office, a social worker, your government representatives, or the National Coalition for Cancer Survivorship.

HOME HEALTH SERVICES

Advances in medicine and technology have made it possible to deliver certain kinds of treatment in the home rather than in hospitals or other facilities. For example, sometimes chemotherapy can be handled by visiting nurses. Physical therapy or nutritional counseling can be provided by in-home therapists. Home health aides can assist with personal care. A skilled nurse can teach you or a member of your family any necessary procedures, such as injecting medications, thus saving trips to the hospital. People who need around-the-clock assistance might consider hiring private-duty nurses, who work in patients' homes all or part of the day.

Other kinds of home care are also available: visits from social workers, sessions with occupational therapists, and meal and transportation services. Independent agencies provide homemaker services, in which a person helps with tasks such as shopping or housecleaning. Some community agencies sponsor visitor programs; volunteers come to a home for regular visits, to provide companionship and conversation. In some areas, a program sponsors ostomy visitors—people who are successfully managing their colostomy and volunteer to make home calls and help others.

Some insurance plans reimburse for home health care expenses only if you are physically disabled and confined to the home or if the services provided are prescribed by a doctor, are short-term, and require a professionally trained caregiver, such as a nurse. Medicare and Medicaid programs do not cover expenses of a private-duty nurse. Ask your insurance provider to explain what services are covered in your policy. Talk to physicians, nurses, social workers, or hospital patient advocates about services available from home health care agencies in your area.

FINANCIAL ASSISTANCE

It goes without saying that treatment for colorectal cancer, especially for recurrent disease, can be expensive. Fear of using up the family's resources is one of the biggest concerns that arises following a diagnosis of cancer. Making matters worse, the disease or its treatment can make it difficult to hold down a job, which poses a risk of loss of income and/or loss of health insurance coverage. Such worries add to the already enormous emotional burden of the disease.

Fortunately, help is available. Hospital financial counselors can help design an installment plan for payments not covered by insurance. Relief for drug costs can be obtained through a variety of programs, including those sponsored by the American Cancer Society and by some drug companies. Social Security and Medicare benefits are available for people over 65 (or, in some cases, 62), and Social Security Disability might apply to some younger people. The Veterans Administration and the American Red Cross provide assistance to men and women who served in the military.

Other forms of government assistance, such as cash grants or food stamps, can also provide relief for low-income families that meet eligibility standards. Many people resist taking advantage of these programs out of a sense of pride or a reluctance to accept charity. It helps to remember that government programs are not charity; they are paid for by tax dollars that came from your pocket. There is no shame or dishonor in taking advantage of programs designed to help people in need.

To find out what's available, talk to your caregivers, especially social workers, and to the credit office of your hospital treatment center. Look in the government pages of the phone book for the names and numbers of relief agencies and the local Social Security Administration office. Talk with your accountant or other financial consultant to learn what medical expenses can be deducted from income taxes.

Many people and families are overwhelmed by the paperwork involved in filing insurance claims and paying medical bills. Some agencies and hospitals may have counselors who can help. Such services are also available for a fee.

NUTRITION

Eating well is a crucial part of recovery from any form of cancer. The body needs a balance of nutrients to function normally, fight off the disease, produce healthy new cells, and recover from the side effects of treatment.

Maintaining a healthy diet while coping with cancer is a challenge. One of the symptoms of cancer is loss of appetite, leading to undesirable weight loss. And side effects from treatment, especially chemotherapy and radiation, can reduce appetite. Some anticancer drugs, for example, produce nausea and vomiting. The disease or its treatment may reduce the body's sense of taste and smell, which lowers interest in eating even further. Depression also produces unhealthy changes in eating habits.

There is no single "cancer diet" that is appropriate for every person. Instead, a diet must be developed that takes individual tastes, preferences, and habits into account, but contains a balance of calories, proteins, vitamins, and minerals. Some dietary supplements can provide nutrients that may be missing from the foods eaten.

A nutritional expert is an important person on any cancer care team. By talking with a professional dietitian soon after your diagnosis, you can pick up tips on how to eat right during and after treatment. For example, experimenting with new types of cuisine or using spices creatively can help stimulate your appetite. Practical strategies, such as eating smaller and more frequent meals, may overcome problems with nausea. A dietitian can also suggest which types of supplements, and in what amounts, might be of benefit. Smart eating will go a long way to prevent future problems that would otherwise interfere with your recovery from colorectal cancer. For more information, see Chapter 11.

ASSISTED LIVING

Every human being wants to live as independently as possible, without having to rely on others or feeling that life has become a burden to self or others. In some cases, however, independent living is not possible, at least until the patient has recovered sufficiently. Options include moving in with a relative or relocating to a rehabilitation center, an assisted living facility, or a nursing home. Such an arrangement can be temporary or permanent. The choice of other living arrangements depends on the person's financial resources and ability to function independently. In any case, relocation can be a profound change in any person's life; it can trigger feelings of loss, sadness, and anxiety, and a sense of fatalism. These "side effects" of cancer must not go unaddressed.

Some patients are able to move into the home of a sibling or an adult son or daughter. But even in the best of circumstances, moving in with a relative can be highly disruptive to everyone's routine. Families may need to take advantage of counseling services to help them adjust to the new reality. Some community or volunteer agencies provide people who will stay with a patient while the family takes a night off or enjoys a much-needed vacation.

HOSPICE CARE

Despite aggressive and effective treatment, many people with colorectal cancer will die from the disease. At some point, it may become clear that further therapy will not produce significant benefit and that death is inevitable. In recent years, the hospice movement has become an important element in compassionate cancer care for the dying.

Hospice care, also known as palliative care, is provided to people whose advanced disease cannot be cured, who are no longer undergoing active therapy, and whose life expectancy can be measured in months rather than years. The goals of palliative care are to control symptoms, prevent suffering, and relieve pain to the greatest degree possible. Hospice care also addresses the physical, emotional, and spiritual needs of the person with cancer as well as the spouse and other members of the family.

In many instances, hospice care can be provided in the person's own home by a team of specially trained professionals. Usually, the team is headed by one or more members of the family who are designated as the primary caregivers. A hospice nurse instructs the family in procedures for administering pain medication, cleaning and changing catheters, providing adequate nutrition, and other necessary steps.

Some hospitals also offer hospice care; in this setting, too, any treatment is aimed not at the disease but at palliation. The number of free-standing residential hospice centers scattered around the country is small but growing. Compared to Europe and other regions, the United States has been slow to embrace the hospice concept, but that situation appears to be changing. Hospice programs that meet certain criteria are covered by Medicare and by some private insurance programs.

Hospice care is not appropriate for everyone with terminal colorectal cancer. In some cases, medical management other than pain relief is needed. Some people with cancer may wish to continue treatment in hopes of achieving a cure, and that is certainly their right. Family members may not be available to carry out the responsibility for around-the-clock care. The decision to begin hospice care should be made only after open and honest discussions among the family and the other members of the health care team. The most important voice, of course, is that of the person with cancer, whose wishes must be respected.

General Tips for Living with Colorectal Cancer

- Think of yourself as a cancer survivor—a person who is *living with cancer.* Continue to take advantage of life's pleasures. The more you feel your life is worth living, the better your life will be.
- Be aware that hiding your diagnosis from others can make you feel isolated and alone. Letting others know about your circumstances opens the door for expressions of love, understanding, and support.
- Keep a diary that records all the medical care you receive for your cancer and for other conditions. These details will be helpful in the years to come as you deal with different doctors and treatment centers.
- Take as much responsibility for your care as you wish to handle. It is your body, and you have the right to determine what treatments and procedures are acceptable to you.
- Be prepared to have other people tell you of their own or their loved ones' experiences with cancer. Resist the temptation to compare your situation with anyone else's. Your case is unique. No two cancers behave exactly the same way. What happened to a "friend of a friend" may not be what happens to you.
- Learn as much as you can about your disease, to reduce your fears and anxieties. Ask your doctor, nurse, or librarian for current information.
- Ask questions if you have trouble understanding something that you read. Write your questions down and bring them to your next appointment. Insist that caregivers explain things in language you can understand. Take notes, bring a tape recorder, or ask a friend or relative to come with you, to help you keep track of what is said. Remember that doctors are busy people. Other personnel in the office, such as the nurse or a physician's assistant, may be willing to give you additional time and information.

- Be aware that family problems that emerge during this time can be the most difficult to handle. Roles change; routines are disrupted; emotions may become ragged. If you and your family can't solve these problems yourselves, consider getting outside help. There is no shame in seeking counseling or support. Not getting help for problems only makes things worse.
- Be prepared to have some friends and acquaintances fade away from your life because they are unable to deal with your situation. By being open and honest about your needs and feelings, you will find other friends—perhaps in surprising places—who can provide the support you need—or a mutual support you can share.
- Reach out and help others. It's one of the best ways to recover emotionally during your fight with cancer. If your strength permits, consider volunteering your time to help others in need.
- Take care of all your needs—physical, emotional, spiritual, and financial.
- Remember that death is the price we pay for being alive, and that death comes to everyone. Don't dwell on thoughts of death, but take practical steps to prepare for it.

BEREAVEMENT COUNSELING

Following the death of a loved one, it is natural—and even healthy—to undergo a process of grieving. Everyone experiences grief in an individual and personal way. Many mourners go through a range of emotions—sadness, anger, fear, guilt, and denial. Some experience physical symptoms, such as loss of appetite, headaches, or trouble sleeping.

There is no right or wrong way to grieve, nor is there any fixed length of time for mourning. The process is different for everyone and depends on the relationship with the deceased, the mourner's personality, and the kinds of support available.

Many people can handle their grief without special assistance, but others may need some help. Talking to someone who is trained in this area may be of benefit. Some social workers, nurses, pastoral counselors, and volunteers are trained as bereavement counselors. Community agencies such as Family Service of America, Catholic Social Services, or Jewish Family Service typically provide support in this area. Hospice programs include grief counseling as part of their care. There are also bereavement support groups whose members have in common the recent loss of a loved one. Private sessions with a professional psychologist or social worker specializing in grief may be helpful. If depression sets in, a physician may suggest a short course of therapy that includes talk sessions and perhaps antidepressant medications.

Adjusting to the death of a loved one can take some time and requires some effort. You may find it comforting to relive memories, wander through old photo albums, and share stories with others touched by the loss. It is normal to experience strong feelings of grief for the first year, as you pass anniversaries, holidays, and other events that remind you of your loss. Often, developing a simple ritual, such as saying a nightly prayer on behalf of the deceased, can help keep your loved one alive in your heart.

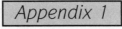
Appendix 1

Staging

As you probably already know, doctors use the concept of *staging* as a way to define the extent of a cancer. A staging system is like a code that gives a quick, consistent description of the problem. The advantage of such a system is that everyone involved in the care of a patient can immediately recognize what the situation is. The type of treatment needed, the outlook, the prospects for survival, and other aspects of cancer care are largely tied to the stage of the disease.

For many people, especially patients and their families caught up in the struggle to understand the diagnosis of colorectal cancer and the treatment options, the staging system can be a little confusing. For one thing, the system—or rather, systems—for defining colorectal cancer continue to change over time. As we learn more about the disease, as treatments keep getting better, we have to keep modifying the system so that it paints an ever-more accurate picture of the clinical reality.

Another factor is that the systems currently available use overlapping but slightly different guidelines for defining the various stages. The definition of a stage varies between colorectal cancer and other forms of cancer, including anal cancer, because different tissues are involved. And while new scientific discoveries are constantly helping us to understand the molecular differences between tumors, it takes some time before those findings can be reflected in staging systems.

One last point: Doctors try to stage cancers as accurately as possible before surgery, but a final staging decision must always wait until after the operation, when a pathologist can study the tissue under a microscope and determine exactly how far the disease has progressed.

With those caveats, then, let's now look at the stages and what they mean.

The first colorectal cancer staging system was named after Cuthbert Dukes, a London physician who published his definitions for rectal cancer stages in 1932. Although other systems are gradually replacing his, you will often hear colorectal cancers

TABLE A1.1: TNM CLASSIFICATION OF COLORECTAL CANCER	
Tx	(No description of the tumor is possible due to incomplete information)
T0	No evidence of primary tumor
Tis	In situ carcinoma; cancer does not penetrate into the submucosa
T1	Tumor invades the submucosa
T2	Tumor invades the main, thickest muscle layers of the colon wall (the muscularis propria)
T3	Tumor invades the subserosa but does not penetrate tissues or organs outside the colon or rectum
T4	Tumor penetrates outside the colon or rectum into neighboring organs or tissues
Nx	(No description of lymph node involvement is possible due to incomplete information)
N0	No lymph node involvement
N1	Cancer cells found in 1 to 3 neighboring lymph nodes
N2	Cancer cells found in 4 or more neighboring lymph nodes
Mx	(No description of metastasis is possible due to incomplete information)
M0	No distant metastasis is found
M1	Distant metastasis is found

Note: Definitions of involved tissues are somewhat simplified.

defined as Dukes' A, Dukes' B, and so on. Other cancers are also frequently described in terms of their ABCD staging, but the word "Dukes" is usually reserved specifically for colorectal cancer.

Over the years, other researchers redefined some of Dukes' original categories. The Astler-Coller system is one example of a modified Dukes' system.

Since the 1980s, however, the system called **TNM**—the system of the American Joint Committee Cancer (AJCC)—has become increasingly accepted for most cancers because it is a more accurate and consistent way of staging many different types of cancers. In this system, **T** stands for the extent of the primary tumor, **N** for the degree of (lymph) node involvement, and **M** for distant metastasis. These letters are each followed by a number that adds details. The higher the number, the more serious the state of each element in the system (see Table A1.1). You may want to glance again at the illustration on page 48 to remind yourself of the names of the tissue layers.

To further simplify these classifications, the American Cancer Society groups various TNM descriptions into five staging categories. See Table A1.2 for these groupings.

TABLE A1.2: STAGE GROUPINGS				
Stage	T	N	M	Explanation
0	Tis	0	0	Carcinoma in situ; cancer in its earliest stages that has not progressed beyond the inner surface of the colon.
I	1 or 2	0	0	Cancer has grown through the lining layer of the colon, but it has not spread outside of the colon wall.
II	3 or 4	0	0	Cancer has grown through the wall of the colon and may have spread into nearby tissue, but it has not spread to the lymph nodes.
III	Any	1 or 2	0	Cancer has metastasized (spread) to nearby lymph nodes, but not to other parts of the body.
IV	Any	Any	1	Cancer has spread to other parts of the body, such as the liver, lung, bone, peritoneum, brain, adrenal glands, or kidney.

TABLE A1.3: COMPARISON OF DUKES' AND TNM STAGES

TNM	TNM Stage	Dukes'	Astler-Coller
Tis	0	—	—
T1-2,N0,M0	I	A	A, B1
T3-4,N0,M0	II	B	B2, B3
T(any), N(1 or 2), M0	III	C	C1, C2, C3
T(any), N(any), M1	IV	—	D

TABLE A1.4: TNM CLASSIFICATION OF ANAL CANCER

Tx	(No description of the tumor is possible due to incomplete information)
T0	No evidence of primary tumor
Tis	In situ carcinoma; cancer does not penetrate into the submucosa
T1	Tumor is 2.0 cm (slightly over 3/4 inch) or less in its greatest dimension
T2	Tumor is larger than 2.0 cm and less than 5.0 cm (2 inches) in dimension
T3	Tumor is larger than 5.0 cm
T4	Tumor of any size invades adjacent organs or tissues
Nx	(No description of lymph node involvement is possible due to incomplete information)
N0	No regional lymph node involvement
N1	Cancer cells found in 1 or more lymph nodes around the rectal area
N2	Cancer cells found in lymph nodes on one side of the pelvis and/or groin
N3	Cancer cells found in lymph nodes at several sites (pelvis or groin nodes on both sides or in rectal area nodes plus pelvis or groin nodes)
Mx	(No description of metastasis is possible due to incomplete information)
M0	No distant metastasis is found
M1	Distant metastasis is found

Put another way:

- Any tumor that has not spread to a lymph node is Stage II or lower.
- Any cancer that involves at least one lymph node is Stage III or higher.
- Any distant metastasis means the cancer is Stage IV.

To see how the TNM system compares with the Dukes' system or as Astler-Coller modified Dukes system, see Table A1.3.

STAGING FOR ANAL CANCER

The staging system for anal cancer is somewhat different than that for colorectal cancer (see Table A1.4).

The definitions for the stage groupings for anal cancer appear in Table A1.5.

Stage	T	N	M	Explanation
0	Tis	0	0	Carcinoma in situ; early cancer that has not spread below the membrane of the first layer of anal tissue.
I	1	0	0	Cancer 2 cm or less that does not involve the sphincter (anal muscle) and that has not spread.
II	2 or 3	0	0	Cancer more than 2 cm that does not involve adjacent lymph nodes or organs.
IIIA	1–3 4	1 0	0	Cancer has spread to lymph nodes around the rectum or to nearby organs.
IIIB	4 Any	1 2 or 3	0	Cancer has spread to lymph nodes in the pelvis or groin on one or both sides, or has spread to adjacent organs and rectal lymph nodes.
IV	Any	Any	1	Cancer has spread to distant lymph nodes within the abdomen or to other organs of the body.

TABLE A1.5: STAGE GROUPINGS

Summary of American Cancer Society Recommendations for Nutrition and Cancer Prevention

1. Choose most of the foods you eat from plant sources.

   Eat five or more servings of fruits and vegetables each day.
   - Include fruits or vegetables in every meal.
   - Choose fruits and vegetables for snacks.

   Eat other foods from plant sources, such as breads, cereals, grain products, rice, pasta, or beans several times each day.
   - Include grain products in every meal.
   - Choose whole grains in preference to processed (refined) grains.
   - Choose beans as an alternative to meat.

2. Limit your intake of high-fat foods, particularly from animal sources.

   Choose foods low in fat.
   - Replace fat-rich foods with foods with fruits, vegetables, grains, and beans.
   - Eat smaller portions of high-fat foods.
   - Choose baked and broiled foods instead of fried foods.
   - Select non-fat and low-fat milk and dairy products.
   - When you eat packaged, snack, convenience, and restaurant foods, choose those low in fat.

Limit consumption of meats, especially high-fat meats.
- When you eat meat, select lean cuts.
- Eat smaller portions of meats.
- Choose beans, seafood, and poultry as an alternative to beef, pork, and lamb.
- Select baked and broiled meats, seafood, and poultry, rather than fried.

3. Be physically active: achieve and maintain a healthy weight.

   Be at least moderately active for 30 minutes or more on most days of the week. Stay within your healthy weight range.

4. Limit consumption of alcoholic beverages, if you drink at all.

   Cancer risk increases with the amount of alcohol consumed and may start to rise with intake of as few as two drinks per day. A drink is defined as 12 ounces of regular remember, 5 ounces of wine, and 1.5 ounces of 80-proof distilled spirits.

COMMON QUESTION ABOUT DIET AND CANCER

Antioxidants

What are antioxidants and what do they have to do with cancer? Certain nutrients in fruits and vegetables appear to protect the body against the oxygen-induced damage to tissues that occurs constantly as a result of normal metabolism. Because such damage is associated with increased cancer risk, antioxidant nutrients are thought to protect against cancer. Antioxidant nutrients include vitamin C, vitamin E, selenium, and carotenoids. Studies suggest that people who eat more fruits and vegetables containing these antioxidants have a lower risk for cancer. Clinical studies of antioxidant supplements, however, have not demonstrated a reduction in cancer risk (see Beta Carotene, Supplements).

Artificial Sweeteners

Do artificial sweeteners cause cancer? Studies of humans have shown no increased risk of cancer from either saccharin or aspartame.

Beta Carotene

Does beta carotene reduce cancer risk? Research has not reproduced the beneficial effects of fruits and vegetables by giving high-dose supplements of beta carotene. For cigarette smokers, such supplements may be harmful.

Bioengineered Foods

What are bioengineered foods, and are they safe? Foods made through techniques of bioengineering or biotechnology have been altered by the addition of genes from plants or other organisms to increase resistance to pests, to retard spoilage, or to improve transportability, flavor, nutrient composition, or other desired qualities. Few such foods have as yet been marketed. At present, there is no reason to believe that these foods will either increase or decrease cancer risk.

Calcium

Is calcium related to cancer? Some research has suggested that foods high in calcium might help reduce the risk of colorectal cancer, but this relationship is not proven. Whether or not calcium intake affects cancer risk, eating foods containing this mineral is important to reduce the risk of osteoporosis. Low-fat and non-fat dairy products are excellent sources of calcium, as are some leafy vegetables and beans.

Carotenoids

What are carotenoids, and do they reduce cancer risk?
Carotenoids are a group of pigments in fruits and vegetables that include alpha carotene, beta carotene, lycopene, lutein, and many other compounds. Consumption of foods containing carotenoids is associated with a reduced cancer risk (see Beta Carotene).

Cholesterol

Does cholesterol in the diet increase cancer risk? There is no evidence that lowing blood cholesterol causes an increase in cancer risk.

Coffee

Does drinking coffee cause cancer? Many studies have found no relationship at all between coffee and the risk of pancreatic, breast, or any other type of cancer.

Cooking Methods

Does cooking affect cancer risk? Some research suggests that frying or charcoal-broiling meats at very high temperatures creates chemicals that might increase cancer risk. Preserving meats by methods involving smoke also increase their content of potentially carcinogenic chemicals. Although these chemicals cause cancer in animal experiments, it is uncertain whether they actually cause cancer in people. Techniques such as braising, steaming, poaching, stewing, and microwaving meats do not produce these chemicals.

Cruciferous Vegetables

What are cruciferous vegetables and are they important in cancer? Cruciferous vegetables belong to the cabbage family, which includes broccoli, cauliflower, and brussels sprouts. These vegetables contain certain chemicals thought to reduce the risk of colorectal cancer.

Fiber

What is dietary fiber and can it prevent cancer? Dietary fiber includes a wide variety of plant carbohydrates that are not digested by humans. Specific categories of fiber are "soluble" (like oat bran) and "insoluble" (like wheat bran). Insoluble fiber is thought to help reduce the risk of colorectal cancer.

Fish Oils

Does eating fish protect against cancer? Fish fats are rich in omega-3 fatty acids. Studies in animals have found that omega-3 fatty acids suppress cancer formation, but there is no direct evidence for protective effect in humans at this time.

Fluorides

Do fluorides cause cancer? Fluorides do not increase cancer risk.

Folic Acid

What is folic acid and can it prevent cancer? Folic acid (sometimes called folate or folacin) is a B vitamin found in many vegetables, beans, fruits, whole grains, and fortified breakfast cereals. Folic acid may reduce the risk of some cancers. Current evidence suggests that to reduce cancer risk, folic acid is best consumed along with the full array of nutrients found in fruits, vegetables, and other foods.

Food Additives

Do food additives cause cancer? No convincing evidence exists that any additive at these levels causes human cancers.

Garlic

Can garlic prevent cancer? Insufficient evidence supports a specific role for this vegetable in cancer prevention.

Genetics

If our genes determine cancer risk, how can diet help prevent cancer? Nutrients and nutritional factors in the diet can protect DNA from being damaged and can delay or prevent the development of cancer even in people with an increased genetic risk for the disease.

Irradiated Foods

Why are foods irradiated, and do irradiated foods cause cancer? Radiation does not remain in the foods after treatment, and there is no evidence that consuming irradiated foods increases cancer risk.

Nitrites

Should I avoid nitrite-preserved meats? Most lunchmeats, hams and hot dogs are preserved with nitrites to maintain color and to prevent contamination with bacteria. Nitrites can be converted to carcinogenic nitrosamines in the stomach, which may increase the risk of gastric cancer. Vitamin C and related compounds are often added to foods to inhibit this conversion. Nitrites in foods are not a significant cause of cancer among Americans.

Olestra

What is olestra and is it related to cancer? Olestra may reduce fat intake, but it also reduces the absorption of fat-soluble carotenes and other potentially cancer-protective phytochemicals in fruit and vegetables. Although reducing absorption substances might also reduce the health benefits of fruits and vegetables, the overall effect of this type of fat substitute on cancer risk is unknown at present.

Olive Oil

Does olive oil affect cancer risk? Consumption of olive oil is not associated with any increase in risk of cancer, and most likely is neutral with respect to cancer risk.

Pesticides and Herbicides

Do pesticides and herbicides on fruits and vegetables cause cancer? Although fruits and vegetables sometimes contain low levels of these chemicals, overwhelming scientific evidence supports the overall health benefits and cancer-protective effects of eating fruits and vegetables. In contrast, current evidence is insufficient to link pesticides in foods with an increased risk of any cancer.

Phytochemicals

What are phytochemicals, and do they reduce cancer risks? The term "phytochemicals" refers to a wide variety of compounds produced by plants. Because consumption of fruits and vegetables reduces cancer risks, researchers are searching for specific compounds in these foods that might account for the beneficial effects. There is no evidence that taking phytochemical supplements is as beneficial as consuming the fruits, vegetables, beans, and grains from which they are extracted.

Salt

Do high levels of salt in the diet increase cancer risk? Little evidence suggests that moderate amounts of salt or salt-preserved foods in the diet effect cancer risk.

Selenium

What is selenium and can it reduce cancer risk? Selenium supplements are not recommended, as there is only a narrow margin between safe and toxic doses. Grain products are good sources of selenium.

Soybeans

Can soybeans reduce cancer risk? Soybeans are an excellent source of protein and a good alternative to meat. Nonfermented soybeans have high levels of phytoestrogens and other phytochemicals that appear to have beneficial effects on hormone-dependent cancers in animal studies. These effects remain to be proven in humans, however.

Supplements

Can nutritional supplements lower cancer risk? Strong evidence associates a diet rich in fruits, vegetables, and other plant foods with reduced risk of cancer, but there is no evidence at this time that supplements can reduce cancer risk.

Tea

Can drinking tea reduce cancer risk? Some researchers have proposed that tea, especially green tea, might protect against cancer because of its content of antioxidants (see Antioxidants). In animal studies, some teas have been shown to reduce cancer risk, but beneficial effects of tea on cancer risk in people are not yet proven.

For Further Reading

Cancer patients, their families and friends, and others may find the following booklets useful. They are available free of charge by calling the American Cancer Society at 1-800-ACS-2345.

- *After Diagnosis: A Guide for Patients and Families.*
  Answers the most common questions about living with cancer.
- *Understanding Chemotherapy.*
  Explains chemotherapy and addresses problems and concerns of patients undergoing this treatment.
- *Understanding Radiation Therapy.*
  Explains radiation therapy and addresses concerns of patients receiving radiation treatment.
- *Taking Time: Support for People with Cancer and the People Who Care About Them.*
  Discusses the emotional side of cancer—how to deal with the disease and to learn to talk with friends, family members, and others about cancer.
- *Caring for the Patient with Cancer at Home.*
  A guide for patients and families.
- *Sexuality and Cancer—Men.*
- *Sexuality and Cancer—Women.*
  Addresses concerns about sexuality facing people with cancer and their partners.

BOOKS ABOUT CANCER

The following list includes some recently published books about cancer generally and about colorectal cancer specifically. Most are available in paperback editions. (This list is offered only as a reference; inclusion here does not constitute endorsement by the author of this book or by the American Cancer Society.)

- *Colon Cancer & the Polyps Connection.* By Stephen Fisher (Fisher Books).
- *Confronting Cancer: How to Care for Today and Tomorrow.* By Michael M. Sherry (Insight Books).
- *Diagnosis: Your Guide Through the First Few Months.* By Wendy Schlessel Harpham, M.D. (W. W. Norton & Co).
- *Informed Decisions: The Complete Book of Cancer Diagnosis, Treatment, and Recovery.* By Gerald P. Murphy, M.D., Lois B. Morris, and Dianne Lange (Viking Press).
- *Prostate Cancer.* By David Bostwick (Villard Books).
- *What to Do If You Get Colon Cancer: A Specialist Helps You Take Charge and Make Informed Choices.* By Paul Miskovitz, M.D., and Marian Betancourt (John Wiley & Sons).
- *A Cancer Survival Almanac: Charting Your Journey.* Nat'l Coalition for Cancer Survivorship (Chronimed Publishing).
- *Share the Care: How to Organize a Group for Someone Who Is Seriously Ill.* By Cappy Capossela and Shelia Warnock (Simon and Shuster).

MAGAZINES, JOURNALS, AND NEWSLETTERS

Hundreds of articles on cancer are published each year. You can locate those that appear in popular magazines and journals in the *Reader's Guide to Periodical Literature,* which is available in most public libraries. If you need help using the guide or finding an article, ask a librarian.

Articles published in over 3,000 health-science journals can be researched in *Index Medicus*. Medical libraries, most colleges and universities, and some public libraries carry this resource.

You can locate cancer-related articles published in health-science journals by using or having access to the National Library of Medicine's (NLM) MEDLARS program. MEDLARS, in turn, provides access to CANCERLIT, a computerized database system which contains almost one million citations and abstracts of articles on cancer from medical and scientific literature.

Librarians in medical libraries and in libraries at nursing schools can retrieve information stored in MEDLARS. However, if you or your doctor want to get information using your own computer system, you can contact NLM at:

MEDLARS Management Section
National Library of Medicine
8600 Rockville Pike
Bethesda, Maryland 20894
(301) 496-6193
(800) 638-8480

Your local library also may be able to do a computer information search. If it belongs to the Federal Library System, you may be able to borrow government publications. You can also do free MEDLINE searches on the Internet. For more information, see the "Resources" section that follow.

Resources

ORGANIZATIONS

American Cancer Society, Inc.
1-800-ACS-2345 (1-800-227-2345)
www.cancer.org
The American Cancer Society is a nationwide community-based voluntary health organization dedicated to eliminating cancer, a major health problem, by preventing cancer, saving lives from cancer, and diminishing suffering from cancer through research, education, advocacy, and service. You can call the ACS National Cancer Information Canter at 1-800-ACS-2345 any time, day or night, 24 hours a day, 7 days a week, to speak with a cancer information specialist about your needs. Spanish-speaking staff is available. Locally available ACS programs include I Can Cope, a series of educational sessions for people facing cancer and Ostomy Rehabilitation visitors for people with ostomies.

Cancer Care, Inc.
1180 Avenue of the Americas
New York, New York 10036
1-800-813-HOPE (1-800-813-4673)
www.cancercareinfo.org
This service arm of the National Cancer Foundation helps patients and families cope with the emotional, psychological, and financial consequences of cancer. Through one-to-one counseling, specialized support groups, educational programs, and telephone, cancer care provides support, guidance, information and referral free of charge.

Cancer Information Service
1-800-4CANCER (1-800-422-6237)
cancernet.nci.nih.gov
The National Cancer Institute sponsors this toll-free number and website. Trained staff members can answer your questions and listen to your concerns. A Spanish-speaking staff is available.

The Concern for Dying
250 West 57th Street
New York, New York 10107
1-212-246-6962
The Concern for Dying is a nonprofit educational organization that distributes information on the living will, a document that records patients' wishes concerning treatment, euthanasia, and death and dying. Psychological and legal counseling are provided, as is referral to local organizations.

Corporate Angel Network
Westchester County Airport, Hangar F
White Plains, New York 10604
1-914-328-1313
www.corpangelnetwork.org
This organization alleviates costs for cancer patients who are receiving special treatment in National Cancer Institute approved treatment centers by arranging for ambulatory patients and one attendant/family member to fly free on corporate aircraft when seats are available.

Hospice Link
Hospice Education Institute
Suite 3-B
190 West Brook Road
Essex, Connecticut 06426-0713
1-800-331-1620 (in Alaska and Connecticut: 1-203-767-1620)

The Hospice Education Institute offers information about hospice care and can refer cancer patients and their families to local hospice programs.

National Association for Home Care
228 Seventh Street, SE
Washington, DC 20003
1-202 547-7424
www.nahc.org
This organization offers information about home care, a list of home care and hospice agencies, and an informative booklet called "How to Select a Home Care Agency."

National Coalition for Cancer Survivorship
1010 Wayne Avenue, Fifth Floor
Silver Spring, Maryland 20910
1-301-650-8868
1-888-937-6227
www.cansearch.org
The National Coalition for Cancer Survivorship is a network of groups and individuals who offer support to cancer survivors and their loved ones. It provides information and resources on support and life after a cancer diagnosis.

National Hospice Organization
Suite 901
1901 North Fort Myer Drive
Arlington, Virginia 22209
1-703-243-5900
Hospice referrals: 1-800-658-8898
www.nho.org
This nonprofit membership organization consists of groups and institutions concerned with or providing care for the terminally ill and their families. The organization furnishes literature,

information, and referrals to local hospice programs and to regional and other national resources.

PDQ Service
The National Cancer Institute has developed PDQ (Physician Data Query), a computerized database designed to give doctors and patients quick and easy access to:

- *The latest treatment information for most types of cancer.*
- *Descriptions of clinical trials that are open for patient entry.*
- *Names of organizations and physicians involved in cancer care.*

Cancer Information Service offices (1-800-4CANCER) provide free PDQ searches. Patients may ask their doctor to use PDQ or may call 1-800-4CANCER themselves. Information specialists at this toll-free number use a variety of sources, including PDQ, to answer questions about cancer prevention, diagnosis, and treatment. The database is available online via the NCI website. For additional written resources about cancer, information about particular forms of the disease, its treatment, and possible side effects, and nutritional information and recipes for the cancer patient, ask the Cancer Information Service to send you information or write:

Office of Cancer Communications
National Cancer Institute Building 31, Room I0A24
Bethesda, Maryland 20892
cancernet.nci.nih.gov

Social Security
1-800-SSA-1213 (1-800-772-1213)
www.ssa.gov
Social Security provides a monthly income for eligible elderly and disabled individuals. Supplemental Security Income (SSI) supplements Social Security payments for individuals who have

qualifying income and asset levels. Medicare is a federal health insurance program for those who receive Social Security benefits. Eligible individuals include those who are 65 or older, people of any age with permanent kidney failure, and disabled people under age 65 who have received Social Security payments for at least 24 months. Call the toll-free number or your local Social Security office to receive information on eligibility for or explanations of coverage, or to apply for any of these programs.

United Ostomy Association, Inc.
19772 MacArthur Blvd.
Suite 200
Irvine, California 92612
1-800-826-0826
www.uoa.org
The United Ostomy Association offers emotional support from others with common problems, although not all members are cancer patients. More than 500 chapters are made up of ostomates whose goal is to provide mutual aid, support, and education to those who have had colostomy, ileostomy, or urostomy surgery.

Veterans Administration (VA)
1-800-827-1000
Eligible veterans and their dependents may receive cancer treatment at a Veterans Administration (VA) Medical Center. Treatment for service-connected conditions is provided, and treatment for other conditions may be available based on financial need.

CANCER INFORMATION ON THE INTERNET

The Internet—a global network of computers all connected by telephone lines—offers a vast library of information, most of it free. The World Wide Web (WWW, or the Web) is a portion of the Internet that allows transmission of pictures and sounds as well as text. Many major organizations concerned about cancer, including the American Cancer Society, have Web sites offering helpful, up-to-date information about the disease and its treatment. You can read this information on your computer screen, or you can download it, save it, and print it out.

Following are some of the major cancer-related Web sites. Be aware that new sites appear daily and old ones expand, move, or disappear entirely. If you don't find what you're looking for, try using one of the Internet search engines (such as AltaVista or Infoseek). These engines are like immense library card catalogs. After you type in the topic you want to find, the engine displays a list of results that might contain what you're looking for. A click of the button and you are connected to that site.

One important caution: The information offered by Web sites, online support groups, or mailing lists can be very helpful, but it varies widely in quality and accuracy. The most reliable sources are major organizations, government agencies, hospitals, or universities, where information is reviewed by noted experts and updated frequently. Less reliable are anecdotal reports or unsubstantiated claims about various therapies. Use good judgment and common sense when evaluating the advice you read in Web sites or mailing list archives. Ask your doctors and caregivers for their opinions of what you find.

- ACOR—Association of Cancer Online Resources (cure .medinfo.org). Links to PDQ statements for both physicians and patients; archives of online discussion groups; connections to many cancer-related information sites on the Web.
- American Cancer Society (www.cancer.org). Information about cancer, including statistics, advice about patient and family counseling, diet, home health care, getting help with medical costs, pain control, prevention, detection, treatment and other subjects. Also, data about local ACS divisions, publications, meetings, programs, events, and links to

other cancer resources on the Web, plus an online form to order selected ACS publications.

- American Gastroenterological Association (www.gastro.org /public.html). Essays and message boards providing information on colorectal cancer and other digestive diseases. Directory for finding gastroenterologists who are members of the American Gastroenterological Association.
- American Medical Association (www.ama_assn.org/aps /amahg.htm) provides a directory of credentials and other information regarding most licensed physicians in the United States.
- Canadian Cancer Society (www.cancer.ca). Facts about cancer, treatment, prevention, and Canadian units of the CCS, in English and French.
- Cancer Guide (http://cancerguide.org/). Information about cancer assembled by a cancer survivor: cancer fundamentals, recommended books, clinical trials, how to research medical literature, alternative therapies.
- CancerWeb (www.graylab.ac.uk/cancerweb.html). From the Cancer Research Trust, a facility in England, a resource listing information aimed at patients or physicians on symptoms, emotional support, personal experiences, and clinical trials. Includes a search engine so you can zero in on specific topics.
- Cansearch: National Coalition for Cancer Survivorship Guide to Cancer Resources (www.cansearch.org). User-friendly guide to Web information, started by a long-term survivor of colon cancer. Overview of sources, information on specific cancers, survivors' stories, and a "Town Hall"— an ongoing, online public discussion among people with cancer.
- CenterWatch Clinical Trials Listing Service (www.center-watch.com/). International listing of current clinical trials, organized by type of disease and, in the case of cancer, by site of the tumor. Also offers information about the researchers

and the medical facilities where the trials are under way, and an electronic mailing list so you can be notified about future studies.

- Center for Alternative Medicine in Cancer Research Center (www.sph.uth.tmc.edu/utcam/). Web site from the University of Texas center, supported by the National Institutes of Health Office of Alternative Medicine, offering detailed summaries of everything currently known about the status of scientific research into alternative, questionable, and unproven therapies, from aloe to shark cartilage.
- Medicine On Line (www.meds.com). Health information service with cancer-related topics (including a section on colorectal cancer), discussion groups, and links to other Web sites.
- MEDLINE Searches from HealthGate (www.healthgate .com/HealthGate/MEDLINE/search.shtml). The U.S. Government maintains a computerized database of millions of medical articles from thousands of international journals. This Web site allows you to search the collection and read or print out the abstracts (summaries) of the articles of interest— all for free. If hard medical data are what you're looking for, this is the place. If you don't understand the articles you find, talk about them with your doctors.
- National Cancer Institute (www.nci.nih.gov). Information for health professions and the public about cancer prevention, detection and treatment including an extensive database of clinical trials.
- National Comprehensive Cancer Center Network (www .nccn.org). A coalition of more than a dozen leading American cancer centers, with information about their treatment guidelines and philosophy, and links to the hospitals' home pages.
- National Institutes of Health (www.nih.gov/). From the U.S. Government, health information, current research, and lists of scientific resources, including a search engine.

- OncoLink (www.oncolink.upenn.edu). Sponsored by the University of Pennsylvania Cancer Center, this excellent Web site offers detailed descriptions of various cancers and medical specialties; news developments; stories by cancer survivors; information about causes and prevention of cancer; current clinical trials; answers to FAQs (Frequently Asked Questions); and information about insurance and financial assistance.
- Quackwatch (www.Quackwatch.com). Provides information about health fraud, including claims regarding cancer treatment.

Internet Mailing Lists

A mailing list is like an online patient support group. People with an interest in the subject subscribe to the list and exchange electronic mail (e-mail) messages. The messages are not private; they are available to everyone. If you wish, you can subscribe and read the messages without ever sending one yourself. You can arrange to have the messages delivered to you as soon as a writer posts one online, or you can ask that the entire day's batch of messages arrive at one time.

To subscribe, send e-mail to the addresses given below. Do not enter any information in the "Subject" line of your message. On the first line of the message, insert the information shown. For the words *your name*, substitute your first and last name, separated by a space. When you no longer wish to take part, you can simply "unsubscribe." These lists are an excellent way to exchange information, ask questions, or just "meet" other people who share similar situations.

CANCER-L (a general support group)
Address: listserv@wvnvm.wvnet.edu
Message: subscribe CANCER-L *your name*

Clinical Trial Finder List
Address: listserv@garcia.com
Message: subscribe ctf *your name*

Clinical Trials Mailing List
Address: majordomo@world.std.com
Message: subscribe Clinical_Trials

Colon Cancer Mailing List
Address: listserv@sjuvm.stjohns.edu
Message: colon *your name*

Another valuable resource is Medinfo.Org (http://cure.medinfo
.org/), which is a central archive containing all of the messages
from all of the cancer mailing lists and discussion groups. You
can browse or search these archives to find answers to specific
questions or to determine whether you would like to subscribe to
the list.

Glossary

Abdomen: The part of the body that contains the stomach, small intestine, appendix, colon, rectum, liver, gallbladder, spleen, pancreas, and kidneys.

Adenocarcinoma: A malignant tumor arising from glandular tissue.

Adenoma: A benign tumor made up of glandular tissue.

Adjuvant chemotherapy: Use of anticancer drugs in addition to initial treatment with surgery or radiation therapy or both.

Analgesic: A drug that relieves pain.

Anastomosis: The reconnection made between healthy sections of the colon or rectum after the cancerous portion has been surgically removed.

Anemia: A condition in which a decreased number of red blood cells may cause symptoms including tiredness, shortness of breath, and weakness. Anemia is often a symptom of cancer, including colorectal cancer.

Anorexia: The loss of appetite.

Antibody: A protein that binds to a specific target on a disease-causing cell or substance and triggers a protective response by the body's immune system. (*See* Antigen.)

Antiemetic agent: A drug that prevents or controls nausea and vomiting.

Antigen: A substance, foreign to the body (such as a bacterium or virus), that stimulates the production of antibodies by the immune system.

Antineoplastic agent: A drug that prevents, kills, or blocks the growth and spread of cancer cells.

Anus: The muscular opening from the rectum to the outside of the body.

Ascending colon: The right-side part of the colon, connected to the small intestine.

Axillary nodes: Lymph nodes found in the armpit (axilla).

Barium enema: The use of a solution (barium sulfate) given by an enema during X-ray examination of the lower intestinal tract. Usually performed as a double contrast barium enema (see separate entry).

Benign: Not harmful; not cancerous.

Benign growth: A swelling or growth that is not cancerous and does not spread from one part of the body to another.

Biological therapy: Modern cancer treatment involving the use of biologicals (substances produced by the body's own cells) or biological response modifiers (substances that affect the patient's defense systems). Immunotherapy is a type of biological therapy.

Biopsy: The removal of a sample of tissue for examination under a microscope to check for signs of a disease such as cancer.

Blood count: The number of red blood cells, white blood cells, and platelets in a sample of blood.

Bowel: The intestine. The large bowel includes the colon and the rectum.

Cancer: general term for more than 100 diseases characterized by abnormal and uncontrolled growth of cells. The resulting mass, or tumor, can invade and destroy surrounding normal tissues. Cancer cells from the tumor can travel (metastasize) through the blood or lymphatic systems to start new cancers in other parts of the body.

Cancer in situ: The stage where the cancer is still confined to the superficial layer of the tissue in which it started.

Carcinoembryonic antigen: see CEA.

Carcinogen: A substance that causes cancer.

Carcinoma: A type of cancer that starts in the skin or the lining of organs. (*See* Adenocarcinoma.)

CEA: Carcinoembryonic antigen; a substance produced by some types of cancerous tumors, including those in the colon and rectum.

CEA assay: A laboratory test measuring the level of carcinoembryonic antigen (CEA). The test is a useful indicator of cancer recurrence following treatment for colorectal cancer.

Chemotherapy: Treatment of cancer using drugs.

Chronic: Persisting over a long period of time.

Chyme: Watery digestive material found in the small intestine and in the first sections of the colon.

Clinical trial: The systematic investigation of the effects of new treatments or therapeutic methods. Clinical trials require formal study plans and involve tests in a human population. In cancer research, a clinical trial generally refers to the evaluation of treatment methods such as surgery, drugs, or radiation techniques, although methods of prevention, detection, or diagnosis also may be the subject of such studies.

Colectomy: An operation to remove all or part of the colon. The surgeon removes the cancerous part of the colon and a zone (called a margin) of surrounding colon as well as some of the mesentary (tissue next to the bowel containing vessels and lymph nodes that might also contain cancer cells). A hemicolectomy is the removal of about half of the colon.

Colon: The long, tubelike organ that removes water from digested food. The remaining material, solid waste called stool, moves through the colon to the rectum and leaves the body through the anus. The colon is sometimes called the large bowel or the large intestine.

Colonoscope: A flexible, lighted instrument used to view the inside of the colon.

Colonoscopy: A procedure to look at the entire colon and rectum through a lighted, flexible tube.

Colorectal: Related to the colon and/or rectum.

Colostomy: A surgical procedure to create an opening between the colon and the outside of the abdomen, allowing discharge of stool into a collection bag attached to the body.

Combination chemotherapy: Use of two or more anticancer drugs.

Combination therapy: Use of two or more modes of treatment, such as surgery, radiotherapy, chemotherapy, or immunotherapy, at the same time or in sequence.

Crohn's disease: A chronic condition that causes inflammation of the intestines; people with extensive Crohn's disease are at higher risk of developing colorectal cancer.

CT scan: A test using computers and X-rays to create images of various parts of the body; sometimes called computed tomography or "CAT" scan.

Descending colon: The left-side section of the colon.

Digestive system: The group of organs that bring food into and out of the body and that metabolize food to extract the nutrients. The digestive system includes the mouth, tongue, saliva glands, esophagus, stomach, liver, gallbladder, pancreas, small intestine, colon, rectum, and anus.

Digital rectal examination (DRE): An exam to detect rectal cancer. The doctor inserts a lubricated, gloved finger into the rectum and feels for abnormal areas.

Double contrast barium enema (DCBE): A diagnostic test for intestinal disease. The colon is filled with a barium solution, most of which is then removed. Air (or carbon dioxide) is then introduced into the intestine to cause the organ to expand, thus permitting a clearer and more revealing X-ray. (*See* Barium enema.)

DRE: Digital rectal examination.

Endoscopy: A procedure for looking through a lighted tube at the inside of body organs or cavities, such as the intestines.

Enterostomal therapist: A health care specialist trained to help patients care for and adjust to their colostomy.

Excision: Surgical removal.

External beam radiation: Radiation therapy delivered by a machine outside the body.

Familial adenomatous polyposis (FAP):   An inherited condition in which several hundred polyps develop in the colon and rectum at an early age. The condition is a severe risk factor for colorectal cancer because some polyps will inevitably progress into cancerous tumors.

Fecal occult blood test (FOBT):   A test to check for hidden (occult) blood in feces.

Feces: Waste matter processed by the colon, stored in the rectum, and expelled from the anus in a bowel movement.

Fiber: The parts of fruits and vegetables that cannot be digested. Also called bulk or roughage. Fiber is an important part of the diet and is helpful in preventing colorectal cancer.

FOBT: Fecal occult blood test.

Gastroenterologist: A doctor who specializes in diagnosing and treating diseases of the digestive system.

Hematuria: Blood in the urine.

Hemoccult (Guaiac) test: Brand name of a test that checks for hidden occult blood in the stool. (See FOBT.)

Hormone: Chemical product of the endocrine glands of the body, which, when secreted into body fluids, has a specific effect on other organs.

Hospice: A concept of supportive care to meet the special needs of patients and family during the terminal stages of illness. The care may be delivered in the home, an inpatient hospice, or a hospital by a specially trained team of professionals.

Ileostomy: A surgical opening in the abdomen connected to the ileum (part of the small intestine). It creates a channel for waste material to leave the body after part of the intestine has been removed. (*See* Colostomy.)

Immune system: The group of organs and cells that defends the body against infection.

Immunotherapy: A type of biological therapy that stimulates the immune system to fight cancer cells more effectively. (*See* Biological therapy.)

Impotence: The inability of a man to have or maintain an erection sufficient for sexual intercourse. Impotence is a possible side effect of rectal cancer surgery. Also known as erectile dysfunction.

Informed consent: The process by which health care providers obtain permission from a patient to perform certain diagnostic tests to administer certain treatments, or to involve that person in a clinical trial or research study.

Infusion: Delivering fluids or medications into the bloodstream over a period of time.

Infusion pump: A device that delivers measured amounts of fluids or medications into the bloodstream over a period of time.

Injection: Pushing a medication into the body with the use of a syringe and needle.

Intestine: One of the digestive organs. The small intestine is a long, narrow tube whose main function is to metabolize food and absorb the nutrients. The large intestine is wider and shorter; its main function is to absorb water and move feces so they can be expelled during a bowel movement.

Intramuscular (IM) injection: An injection of medication directly into the muscle.

Intraperitoneal: Within the peritoneal cavity, the area that contains the abdominal organs.

Intravenous (IV) injection: An injection of medication into the vein.

Investigational new drug: A drug that is approved by the U.S. Food and Drug Administration (FDA) for use in clinical trials but has not yet been approved for sale.

Investigator: Clinical researcher studying a new drug or treatment method.

Laparoscopy: A procedure for looking inside the abdominal cavity through a lighted tube.

Lesion: A lump or abscess that may be caused by injury or by a disease such as cancer.

Local therapy: Treatment that affects only a tumor and the area close to it.

Localized tumor: A cancerous growth that has not metastasized to distant parts of the body.

Lower GI series: A series of X-rays of the colon and rectum that is taken after the patient is given a barium enema. GI stands for gastrointestinal. (*See* Barium enema.)

Lymph: The nearly colorless fluid that travels through the lymphatic system and carries cells that help fight infection and disease.

Lymph nodes: Hundreds of bean-sized collections of immune system cells that serve as filters to remove waste products. The lymph nodes trap cancer cells or bacteria that are traveling through the body in lymph. In most cases, colorectal cancer tumors first metastasize to lymph nodes. (Also called the lymph glands.)

Lymphatic system: A network in the body that includes the lymph nodes, lymph fluid, and lymphatic vessels, and, in the broadest sense, the bone marrow, spleen, and thymus. The lymphatic system produces and stores cells that fight infection and disease and serves as a filtering system for tissue fluids.

Lymphedema: Swelling due to blockage of lymph fluid causing fluid retention in a particular part of the body such as the arms or legs. Removal or radiation therapy of lymph nodes can cause lymphedema.

Lymphoma: A cancer of the lymphatic system.

Malignant: Cancerous; malignant cells can spread to (invade) nearby tissues and travel (metastasize) to other parts of the body.

Malignant tumor: A tumor made up of cancer cells that can spread to other parts of the body. (*See* Benign tumor.)

Medical oncologist: A doctor who specializes in treatment of cancer using medications.

Metastasis: The migration of cancer cells from the original tumor site (primary cancer) through the blood and lymph vessels to produce cancers in other tissues. A secondary cancer growing at a distant site is also called a metastasis.

Metastasize: To travel from the original cancer site.

Metastatic cancer: Cancer that has spread from its original site to one or more additional body sites.

Monoclonal antibodies: Artificially manufactured antibodies designed to circulate in the body and attach to targets on cancer cells. Antibodies can be used diagnostically to reveal hard-to-spot tumors, or they can be made to carry anti-cancer treatments such as drugs or radiation directly to the cancerous cells.

MRI (magnetic resonance imaging):   A test that provides in-depth images of organs and structures in the body.

Mucosa: The lining layer of certain organs such as those of the mouth and gastrointestinal tract. Also known as mucous membrane.

Mucus: The fluid produced by a mucous membrane.

Neoplasm: A new growth of tissue or cells; can refer to a benign tumor or a malignant tumor.

OCN (oncology certified nurse):   A registered nurse who has met the training requirements and has successfully completed a certification examination in oncology.

Oncologist: A doctor who specializes in treating cancer.

Oncology: The study and treatment of cancer.

Oncology clinical nurse specialist: A registered nurse with a master's degree who specializes in the education and treatment of cancer patients.

Ostomy: An operation to create an opening from an area inside the body to the outside. (*See* Colostomy; Ileostomy.)

Palliative treatment: Treatment aimed at the relief of pain and other symptoms but not intended to cure the disease.

Pathologist: A doctor who identifies diseases by studying cells, tissues, and body fluids under a microscope or by other laboratory tests.

Pathology: The study of disease by the examination of tissues, cells, and body fluids.

PDQ: Physicians Data Query. A computerized database containing information about cancer treatment, sponsored by the National Cancer Institute and available to physicians nationwide. A simplified version of the same information is also available to patients and lay readers.

Placebo: An inert substance sometimes used in clinical trials for comparison.

Polyp: A growth of tissue protruding into a body cavity, such as a nasal or rectal polyp. Polyps may be benign or malignant.

Primary tumor: The original cancer site.

Prognosis: The projected outcome or course of a disease; the patient's chance of recovery.

Protocol: The outline or plan for use of a procedure or experimental treatment; a clinical trial is designed to test the effectiveness of an experimental protocol.

Radiation oncologist: *See* Radiologist.

Radiation therapy (also called radiotherapy): Treatment using X-rays, protons, electrons, neutrons, or other types of radiation to kill cancer cells.

Radiologist: A doctor who specializes in the use of radiation to diagnose disease (a diagnostic radiologist) or to treat cancer (a radiation oncologist).

Radiosensitizers: Drugs that can boost the effectiveness of radiation therapy.

Randomized clinical trial: A study in which patients with similar traits, such as extent of disease, are placed randomly in separate groups to compare different treatments.

Rectum: The last six to eight inches of the large intestine. The rectum stores solid waste until it leaves the body through the anus.

Recurrence: The reappearance of a cancer after a period of remission.

Regression: Shrinkage of a cancerous growth, usually as a result of treatment.

Relapse: The reappearance of a disease such as cancer in a patient after a period of remission.

Remission: The decrease or disappearance of evidence of a disease; also, the period during which this occurs. Remission can be temporary or permanent.

Resection: Surgical procedure to remove all or part of a diseased or injured organ.

Risk factor: Anything that increases a person's chances of developing cancer. Familial adenomatous polyposis is a risk factor for colorectal cancer.

Side effect: A secondary and usually unwanted effect from a drug or other treatment. Side effects result from the impact of treatment on healthy cells. Common side effects of cancer treatment are fatigue, nausea, vomiting, decreased blood cell counts, hair loss, and mouth sores.

Sigmoid colon: The S-shaped part of the colon between the descending (left) colon and the rectum.

Sigmoidoscope: A lighted instrument used to view the inside of the lower colon. (*See* Colonoscope.)

Sigmoidoscopy: An examination of the rectum and lower colon using a sigmoidoscope. Also called proctosigmoidoscopy or flexible sigmoidoscopy. (*See* Colonoscopy.)

Staging: A system for establishing the extent of a patient's disease.

Standard treatment: An accepted form of therapy that past studies have proved to be of clear benefit.

Stoma: An artificial opening between two cavities or between a cavity and the surface of the body.

Stool: Feces; the solid matter discharged in a bowel movement.

Surgery: An operation.

Systemic: Affecting the entire body.

Systemic therapy: Treatment that reaches cells throughout the body by traveling through the bloodstream.

Taste alteration: A temporary change in taste perception.

Therapeutic: Pertaining to treatment.

Tissue: A group or layer of cells that performs a specific function.

Transverse colon: The horizontal section of the colon.

Tumor: An abnormal overgrowth of cells. Tumors can be either benign or malignant.

Ulcerative colitis: A disease that causes long-term inflammation of the lining of the colon. People with colitis are at higher risk of developing colorectal cancer.

Ultrasonography: A test in which sound waves (ultrasound) are bounced off tissues and the echoes are converted into a picture (sonogram). Also known as *Ultrasound examination.*

X-ray: High-energy radiation used in low doses to diagnose cancer and in high doses to treat cancer.

Index

internal radiation, 146
Internet, information resources
    on, 244–248
intestines, function of, 7
intraoperative radiation, 146
irradiated foods, 233
irritable bowel syndrome,
    109–110

J

jejunum, 12

L

lamina propria, 25
laparoscopy, 133–135
large bowel, function of, 7
large intestine:
    function of, 20–23
    surgical treatment of, 122–125
laser surgery, 126
left radical hemicolectomy, 129
leucovorin, 144–145
levamisole, 143–144
lifestyle, implications of, 55, 83
liver tumors, 132
local excision, 126
local full thickness resection,
    126
loop colostomy, 204
low anterior resection, 131
lunch, sample menus, 173–174
lungs:
    cancer of, 10–11
    metastases, 109
lymphatic system, 25–26
lymph nodes, 51

M

macrobiotic diet, 161
magnetic resonance imaging
    (MRI), 118
malignant tumors, 31, 49–50
Medicare/Medicaid, 215
Medicine On Line, 246
MEDLARS, 237–238
MEDLINE, 238, 246–247
mesentery, 128
metabolism, 53
metastasis:
    defined, 7
    diagnosis and, 108–109
    implications of, generally,
      31–32
metastasized cancer, surgical
    treatment of, 124, 132
metastates, 108–109
metastatic adenocarcinomas, 50
metastatic cancer, 32
mineral supplements, 63, 68
mitomycin, 148
morphine, 155
mucosa, 24
mucosal glands, 25
mucous membrane, 24
muscle cells, 27
muscularis mucosae, 25

N

napkin ring effect, 107
National Association for Home
    Care, 240
National Cancer Institute, 172, 247
    Cancer Information Service,
      208–209

National Coalition for Cancer
Survivorship, 240
National Comprehensive Cancer
Center Network, 247
National Hospice Organization,
242
National Institutes of Health,
159, 247
National Public Health Institute
of Finland, 82
neoadjuvant therapy, 142
nitrites, 233
NSAIDs:
effectiveness of, 75–76
impact of, 75
for pain control, 156
prostaglandins, 74–75, 77
side effects, 76
sulindac, 77–78
nutrition, American Cancer
Society recommendations
for, 228–235
nutritional therapy, 172

O

obesity, 38
obstruction, 107, 108
occupation, as risk factor, 38–39
Office of Alternative Medicine
(OAM), 159
Office of Cancer
Communications, 243
olestra, 233–234
olive oil, 234
oltipraz, 84
OncoLink, 247
Oncology Nursing Society, 88

open-ended support groups, 207
open surgery, 133–135
Ostomy Rehabilitation Program,
242
ovarian cancer, 83

P

pain:
abdominal, 10, 34–35, 106,
108–109
control, 155–157
palliative care, 219
palliative surgery, 126, 132–133
palliative therapy, 146–147
Papillon technique, 146
paradoxical diarrhea, 108
PDQ Service, 242–243
pedunculated polyps, 47
peer counselors, 207
perforation, 135, 138
pesticides, 234
PGE2, 78
Physician's Health Study, 81
phytochemicals, 63, 234
piroxicam, 77
polypectomy, 32, 49, 116
polyposis, defined, 40
polyps, see Adenomas
benign, 45
bleeding and, 92
development of, 31
growth of, 5
implications of, 4
in large intestine, 8
malignant, 47
noncancerous, 87
pedunculated, 47

About the Author

In 1994, BERNARD LEVIN, M.D., was appointed the first full-time vice president for cancer prevention at the University of Texas M. D. Anderson Cancer Center, and he is still serving in this capacity today. He earned his medical degree from the University of the Witwatersrand Medical School in Johannesburg, South Africa, as well as completing his surgical and medical internships there. Later, at the University of Chicago, he completed an internal medicine residency, a research fellowship in biochemistry in pathology, and a clinical fellowship in gastroenterology. After several academic appointments at the University of Chicago, he was named chairman of the Department of Gastrointestinal Medical Oncology and Digestive Diseases. Currently, he is chair of the American Cancer Society's National Advisory Task Force on Colorectal Cancer, a member of the American Gastroenterologoical Association, a fellow of the American College of Physicians, and a consultant to the National Cancer Institute.

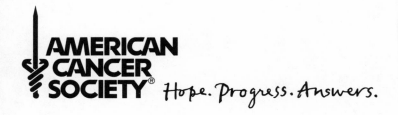

AMERICAN CANCER SOCIETY® *Hope. Progress. Answers.*

The American Cancer Society is the nationwide community-based voluntary health organization dedicated to eliminating cancer as a major health problem by preventing cancer, saving lives from cancer, and diminishing suffering from cancer through research, education, and service.

For information on cancer and on American Cancer Society educational programs and services, please contact:

Toll-free cancer information: 1-800-ACS-2345
Home page address: http://www.cancer.org